Dirty Sex Talk:

How to Talk Dirty, Reveal Your Secrets. The Guide to Seduce for Woman and Men, Overcomes the Taboo with Examples. Sex for Women and Men.

by Paula Ann & Damian Old

Table of Contents

Chapter 5 Dirty Talk Phrases To Get You Started............57

Chapter 6 Sensuous Seduction...94

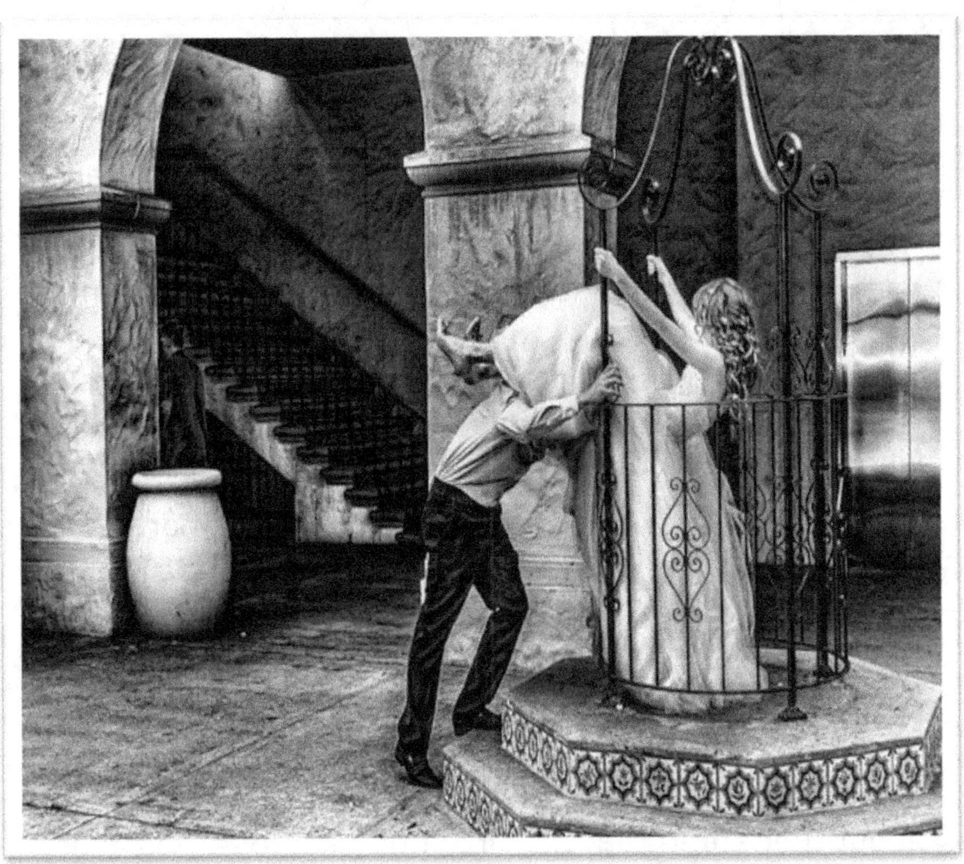

Introduction

The mind is a beautiful thing and as it turns out, an untapped reserve packed with sensual stimuli waiting to be awakened. One right word is all it takes to heighten your lover's arousal. One right word uttered at the right time can increase the intensity of the orgasms you have. But mention the words "dirty talk" and many couples immediately put their guard up and back away from the subject, treating it as something shameful that should not be discussed. Why? Why continue to suppress that primal side of our nature when it could lead to the source of our greatest physical pleasure? Why do we continue to ignore the power that these words have to help us become the wild lovers we secretly long to be?

For too long, dirty talk has been treated as something shameful that many couples are reluctant to talk about. For some reason, dirty talk has got a bad rep for itself over the years as "cheap" talk that only prostitutes and porn stars would resort to. Nothing could be further from the truth. If you've tried everything to get closer to your partner's raw emotions and increase the intimacy between the sheets but always seem to fall short, that's because you haven't tried dirty talk. Once you get over the fear of being rejected or judged for your less than honorable fantasies, you will see how beneficial this talk can be for your sex life.

The truth is, dirty talk can skyrocket your sex life in a way nothing else can. Not even the kinkiest toys or the nastiest moves can provide the same experience you get when you learn to verbalize the naughty thoughts and desires you've kept buried in your mind for so long. It certainly looks like you're ready to take your relationship to new heights since you're here now with a copy of this book.

There is a world of difference between pillow talk and dirty talk. Pillow talk may or may not lead to sex and usually doesn't take place during sex. It happens before or after sex and focuses on emotional intimacy. Dirty talk, on the other hand, is raunchy, sexually charged, sexually explicit, and more focused on enhancing the act of sex.

Discussing the things, you like about your partner, sharing your dreams, fears, and special memories (which are all examples of pillow talk) can make couples feel very close. Still, people can be emotionally intimate, yet have boring sex. To up your physical intimacy game, you need to say and hear the things that step you up from being emotionally intimate with your partner to feel like devouring them in bed! Dirty talk allows you to freely express yourself to your sexual partner – telling them what you want and also learning what they fantasize about or prefer.

The feeling of love is essential in relationships, but most people don't just want to feel loved. They want to feel wanted, desired, and lusted after. Dirty talk brings all that feeling to life. Spicing up your romantic or sexual relationship doesn't have to be hard work. You don't need extra tools and props to make your sex life more exciting. You already possess all the essential tools to turn up the passion in your sexual relationship. Vocalizing what you want and what you want to do is one of those tools. If done correctly, dirty talk can even be more exciting than the actual act of physical sex. One of the biggest challenges for many people is bypassing their conception of dirty talk. After all, what good can there be in something gross, filthy, and even profane? Perhaps, a simple way to overcome the idea of "dirty" would be to tweak the term "dirty talk" to read "the power of words." Think of this book as a guide to using the power of words to spice up your sex life.

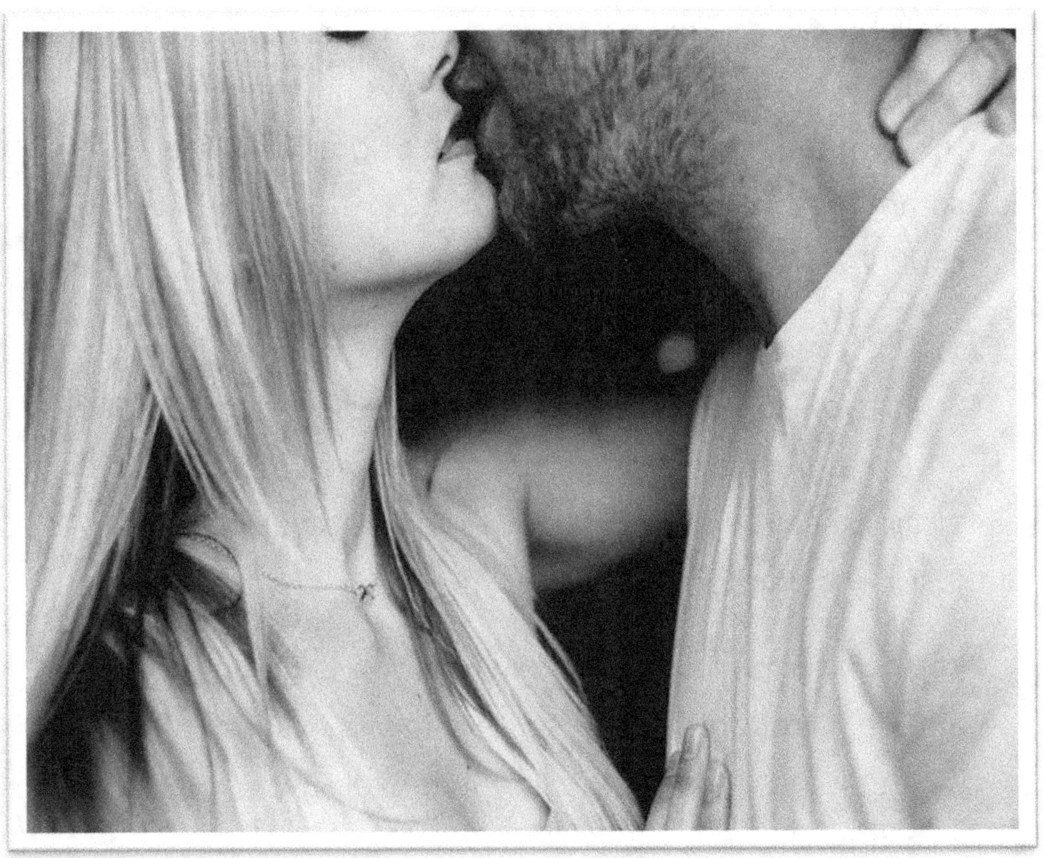

Chapter 1 Why, When, How To Use Dirty Talk With Your Partner

Most girls often like it, but very few speak dirtyly to their boyfriends or husbands during sex. The main problem girls have in this area is to find the words they want to use, but I have a solution. Here are some tips I have collected from a user forum that could help you start and talk perfectly dirty.

1. Tell your man what he wants you to do and how he wants you to do that, but don't be too sweet about it. It's all about being frank, open and free, don't be afraid to say' fuck me dad' or' my juicy wet pussy is just punching for you.'

You don't know how this conversation is going to turn him on. Although it may seem odd the first few times, it can be learned by practice, just like anything else in a relationship.

2. Begin with the fundamentals. It feels like a whole new experience every time I have sex with my boyfriend because each time we start with the basics.

He might be asking me what I wear, and I'll not answer anything or lingerie (even when I'm not), and I'll ask him what he'd do to me if he put his hands on me. This might take a while. Remember that dirty talk does not start in bed, it's a cycle that even before seduction starts.

3. Ask him what you want him to do, but just make it simple and rational. For example, you can tell him to kiss you or tighten you, but don't forget to keep a voice.

Men are creatures who like challenges and challenge him not to do anything that will boost his confidence and make him want. Nevertheless, remember to pay credit for where you owe it if he does something that makes you feel good to say that.

4. Visualize what you mean when you explain how you feel about him. Because sex means emotions, this is what you should focus on when you dirty talk. He may not see or hear what you are feeling, however, and it is up to you to say it in words and actions.

Inform him about the trembling of your back and tell him how your hard cock felt in your cunt, how amazing it feels to have your tongue-everything builds what can be considered refined dirty speech strategies during sex.

5. Did you try to be thematic when you dirty talk? This is especially great if you play a role. For example, you might be a lady and he would be a gentlemen, and dirty talking would go like "Excuse me sir, you might be kind enough to penetrate my vagina with your huge member?

Nonetheless, the theme is based on the early stages of pregnancy, and the better if you can hold it through the session. The prostitutes and the trick when you want it, pirates, the teacher and pupil, the instructor and the cheerleader and others are the most common topics.

There is no script to follow when you speak dirty, it is only one of the personal stuff that two people learn over time. You should know how, what to do and what your man wants to hear or responds to when you solve the initial problems.

I hope these 5 points help you continue your unfriendly yet enjoyable sex life and ultimately strengthen your relationship.

5 Step Guide That You Can Follow To Dirty Talk Properly

One of the warmest and easiest ways to spice up your love life and make sex something completely new is to dirty talk.

Many girls like to test their dirty talk in their bedroom, but their biggest obstacle often is their fear-the fear of their boyfriends or husbands reacting, the fear of not knowing what to say, of embarrassment and unpleasant reactions and the biggest-of not knowing what to say.

Here is a 5-step guide you should follow to dirty talk and always make the experience something for you and your family.

Step 1: Begin with a narrative form of dirty talking

The easiest way to dirty talk is through storytelling, particularly when you are not sure what to say. One of those five things can be described as a narrative of dirt speech:

a) What you will do

(b) What is going on with you

(c) What you are doing

(d) What you feel like

(e) What you want to do with you

Step 2: Sexy Answers

You can begin to practice sexy responses even before you get to the real sex-say, when you speak, flirt or talk publicly. If your partner asks for something like' Do you like that,' instead of a straightforward'

Yeah! It's heaven in me, please, you can speak. It is important to note that your answers should be short, honest and constructive.

Step 3: Hot questions

Consider spicing sex with fun questions if you have a friend who is more passive than you are. Your questions are constructive and should not be difficult to answer. Good examples of sexy questions are:'

Will you like this child?

Is that what you would like?'

And' Am I right, sweetheart?

Step 4: Play with new phrases and sounds

A big part of dirty talking is special, and that is your naively and practice. This is also smart, because you're not going to risk seeing what he saw in porn films. Make it all new-sighs, rumblings, moans, heavy breathing and talking.

Step 5: Study your man

You will know with time which words or terms are turning him off and which ones are doing what you want. Together with the noises you make and the things you say, do what makes him crazy. You should know that sex is not the same dull routine, but a fiery experience that continues to improve as you learn new phrases and acts.

Every woman will admit that one very important thing in a relationship that cannot be compromised is sex. Each man also will admit that they are prepared to do nearly anything to ensure that marriage or the partnership lasts forever so long as their sex lives are decent.

The biggest challenge, though, is to get rid of the monotony of most intimate relationships and marriages. In fact, the answer is very simple: to dirty talk during sex. Though dirty talk is very popular, not all girls know how to do it correctly. Some fire it once or twice and give it all up if it gets awkward or humiliating.

I have some ideas to help you learn what dirty talk really is and how to do it correctly. The first piece of information I can give you is to find the right sources. Don't just listen and blindly follow what your girlfriends say.

Sexologists and sex therapists with extensive experience in these topics have created some excellent eBooks and guides, you will consider one. The trick to understanding and perfecting how to dirty talk is to understand what it really is and to follow the right steps or guides.

You will figure out what your man likes and doesn't like, because men are special. If you're a shy girl, you certainly can start with simple words and flirtatious messages. You can build atmosphere while your man is away by sending him sexy messages and flirting over his mobile.

That, if it goes well, will set the stage for good sex, open communication lines and help you build confidence. When it comes to sex, this is where you have to call the inner slut up.

There are various kinds of sentences you can use. The best start would be to tell your husband how you feel and dig up your body's thoughts and emotions. The other way of dirty talking is by telling him what you want him to do-how you spit, squeeze the nipples or whisper to your ear. The third way of dirty talk is to tell your husband and ask what he's doing well.

Each man wants an unpredictable woman who is willing to try different things to make her relationship and particularly her sex life happier and exciting. You're this type of girl?

I'm sure you're glad you read this. I have a few suggestions that, I'm sure, will motivate you to learn to dirty talk in bed and make sex a whole new experience with your boyfriend.

a) Idea analysis. You're already looking for ideas, that are good. Once you read other women ' posts, opinions and ideas, you will get a better idea of what dirty talking is. The notion of dirty talk would most girls dismiss as something for sluts and porn stars, but is that not just what a man wants in bed?

b) Get a manual for directions. The best thing you can do to avoid anything getting mixed is to find a full guide, such as an eBook, written by someone that has sex and dirty talk experience. Such an eBook will have all the details you need when you master the baby steps of dirty talking in bed.

c) Quick launch. The best place to begin is to moan and whisper sweet words in your ear. You can't just start screaming and shouting, because this can be a mood killer, and it is unnatural and fake. Saying words like "I'm feeling good" and "oh yes! "It's sufficient to change what he feels and does.

d) Practice what you're looking for. You can play in your bathroom with the words you have stored in your head while you "alone" and even use them when you are flirting or sexting. Dirty talk is a mixture of many aspects that you often know with the time.

Know your guy well. Know your man well. He doesn't want any words or phrases, know what they are and stop them. Know what sentences to turn on him and know when to use them. Practice the sentences you use to tell him how you feel, what he needs to do and what he has done correctly. While it may be odd and awkward to dirty talk the first few times, you will see with time how good it is for a relationship. Use these top 5 tips to change your sex life completely starting tonight!

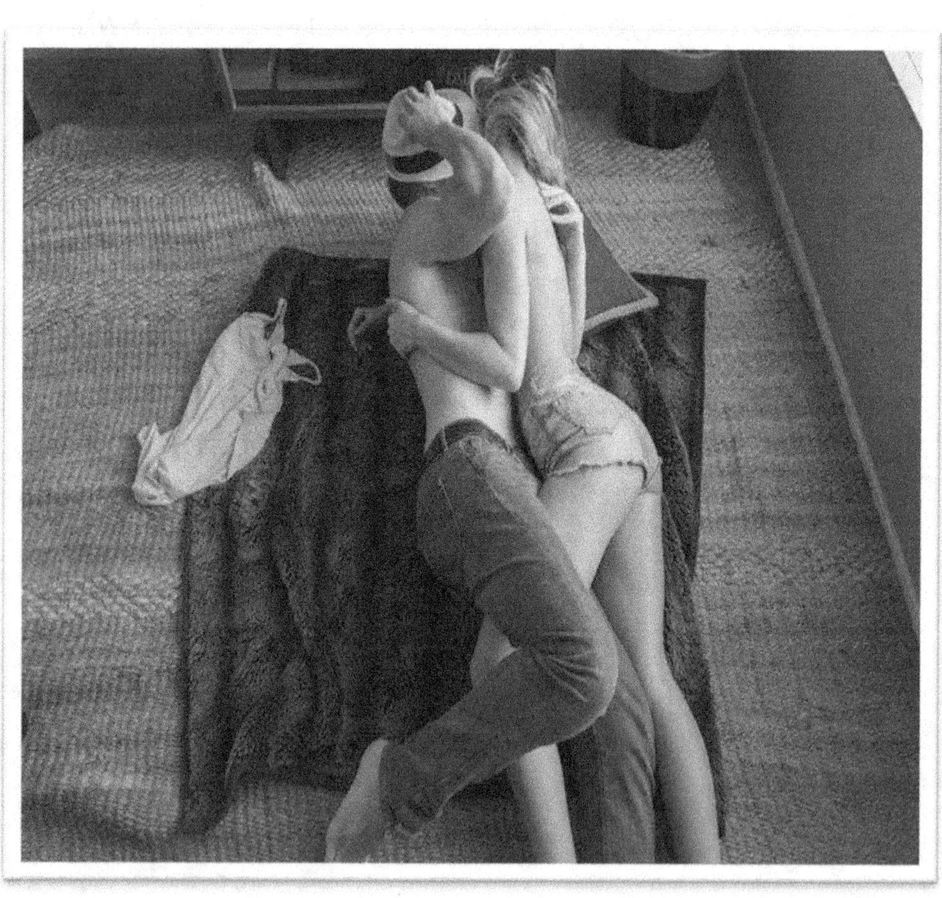

Chapter 2 How Dirty Talk Will Free Your Inhibitions

You'll never know what it's like to free your sexual inhibitions until you've dirty talked your way to sex so mind-blowing it leaves you both panting and gasping after it's done. There's an inner sexual animal within all of us that is waiting to be released, and when we let go of the taboos and the mental chains that weigh us down, there's an indescribable sexual experience that awaits.

But I've never tried dirty talk before. Where would I even begin? Let's start at the beginning with the types of dirty talk options you have and how to work your way past the shy, uncomfortable phase so it starts to feel natural. After all, the whole point is to kick your sex drive up a few notches, and the last thing you want is to feel like it is nothing but a painful, cringe-worthy encounter.

The Different Types of Dirty Talk

Sex positions are not the only thing that comes with options. As it turns out, dirty talk does too. Well, you've got two options to work with at least:

• Softcore Dirty Talk - Otherwise known as the "sweet nothings" you sometimes whisper in your partner's ear. The language used in this variation is not exactly what you would call "dirty". In fact, softcore dirty talk actually sounds warm, affectionate, and even encouraging at times. The purpose of this type of talk is to try and entice your partner's feelings and play on their affection for you to get them in the mood. If you're just starting out in the dirty talk arena, then softcore is the way to go when you're trying to gauge the way your partner feels about it. This is an experience you've probably never attempted before, and as with introducing anything new, it's best to go slow and test the waters instead of coming in full force with the X-rated talk and catch your partner off guard. Some examples of what this type of dirty talk would sound like include: You're the sexiest thing I've never seen. I want you so badly right now. You have no idea what I want to do to you with my tongue and fingers. Don't be fooled by how lukewarm they sound though, the secret to making it work is in the way that you say it. Say it passionately, say it aggressively, say it with lust, desire, through clenched teeth like you can't control your urges any longer, and say it in a low, gruff voice that shows your partner you're having a hard time trying to control yourself from ravaging them. To amp it up, softcore talk sounds even sexier when you're looking at your partner's body or genitals instead of their face.

•	Hardcore Dirty Talk - These can be quite intimidating if you've never attempted to use them before since hardcore talk tends to be direct and sometimes even vulgar. Hardcore dirty talk is best used when you're trying to trigger a physical response out of your partner instead of an emotional one. This type of talk is meant to appeal to our innermost primal, animal instinct. Think hardcore, full-on, bed-shaking sex since this talk is meant to encourage the animal within us to come out. Partner's need to drop their inhibitions with hardcore talk and let it all go so they can completely surrender to the pleasure that awaits. In the hardcore talk, expect the use of swear words every now and again. Profanity and sexy are probably two words you would never think of using in the same sentence, but when swear words slip out during your lovemaking, it gives the impression that you're losing control and indicates to your partner that the sex is so incredible you're at a loss for words how to describe it. Some couples use hardcore dirty talk to push their boundaries as they attempt to recreate their sexual fantasies and make the role play appear more realistic. Imagine you were playing the role of the "innocent" next-door neighbor for example. In this role, you're supposedly naive and innocent, and the thought of any kind of profanity escaping your lips is unheard of. Therefore, when it comes out during your vigorous lovemaking, it's like your character is breaking all the rules and giving in to their animal lusts, which your partner could find an incredible turn on. One of the biggest advantages of this talk is how raw and honest it feels. Oh yes, you feel so hard inside me. I'm going to make your gorgeous tits bounce so hard when I'm pounding you. Put your cock inside me, baby, I want to scream as you fill me up. The key is hardcore talk is to use words that you and your partner are comfortable using. If using words like tits, pussy, fuck, or cock don't feel right, you don't have to force yourself to use it. This is supposed to feel natural, so say whatever comes to mind in the heat of the moment.

Types of Dirty Talk

Getting Over the Awkward Hump

The best sexual conversations happen when we keep it simple, honest, and straightforward. Dirty talk doesn't have to be difficult, not unless you wanted it to be. You know what you want. You tell your partner what you want. You know what you would like to do. You tell your partner what you're going to do. That's all there is to that dynamic. Honest. Straightforward. To the point. Yet, despite the simplicity, many people still freeze and find themselves stuck when it's showtime. It's not that they don't want to do it. They just feel weird about it and they don't know how to get past that.

If it feels weird and uncomfortable, you might be wondering why should I bother dirty talking at all? Isn't it better to just keep things the way they are? You could, but if there was even the slightest possibility that you could skyrocket your sexual pleasure, wouldn't you want to give it a go at least? Once you've experienced game-changing sex, it is never going to be the same again. Sex is an overall mind and body experience, and if your body is feeling something but your mind is disengaged, no matter how hard you or your partner try, you're still going to fall short of sexual nirvana. Dirty talk is one way of coaxing yourself and your partner out of your own heads. Anything new is always going to feel strange in the beginning, but once you get past the initial awkward stage, it's only going to be smooth sailing from that point onwards. Yes, it is possible to dirty talk without feeling foolish, and here's how you do it:

• Keep It Simple - You don't need to go all out right from the start, despite what the porn videos you might have watch tried to tell you. You and your partner have a rhythm and a dynamic between you that works, and that's the strength you should capitalize on. Instead of trying too hard to make it perfect, start slow and keep it simple by going with what feels the most natural at the time. There's no need to construct an over-the-top, elaborate sex script before you hit the sheets. Dirty talk isn't supposed to sound rehearse, it should stem from the emotions you feel in the heat of the moment. If starting with something simple like I can't wait to rip your clothes off and feel how hard you are inside me is good enough to get the momentum going. Don't feel pressured right away to use words you haven't used before, it's okay if you need time to work up to it. Keep it simple and playful in the beginning.

•   Be the Coach - There are two ways you can approach your dirty talk encounter. The first is to use it to build anticipation. The second is to take on the role of the "coach" or "director" who instructs your partner what to do. If you're used to giving instructions in your job, this one is a pretty easy concept to transfer into the bedroom. The right amount of instruction can be something your partner may find a turn on. An example of what this might look like is: Put on that sexy black lingerie of yours that I like tonight and lie down on the bed. I'm going to do things to you that will make you scream.

•   Talk Dirty When You're Not Having Sex - Practice makes perfect, and if you're struggling with getting over "how weird" dirty talk feels, this might help with that. Couples who are comfortable talking about their sex lives tend to have greater satisfaction in that department. Most of the time, people feel intimidated by the idea of dirty talk because they have no idea what to say or how to say it. They feel tongue-tied when it's time to step up and do it. Which is where the practice bit comes in handy. When you're comfortable talking about sex in everyday conversation, you eventually get comfortable with the terminology and the sexual innuendos involved so it doesn't seem to awkward anymore when it's time to turn the conversation "dirty".

•   Learn to Talk About It - Expect a few bumps and slip-ups along the way when you're new to this whole experience. There could be a time or two when you say something that rubs your partner the wrong way, even if they might not say it out loud, you can sense a shift in the mood. Should you feel like you may have taken things a step too far, it is important to communicate and talk to each other about it. For example, some couples might get turned on calling their partner "daddy" in bed because of the sexual dominance associated with it. But that might not be something your partner is comfortable with. To them, it might have incestuous connotations and that ends up ruining the moment. Talk to your partner about what works and what doesn't. Ask them what words trigger their fantasies and let them know what yours are. It's important that you learn to talk about the difficult parts of the process together so you're both on the same page about it.

•   Talk About What You're Doing - Say what you're doing, what you want to do, and how you're going to do it. That's the easiest way to start dirty talking if you're struggling to know where to begin. Tell your partner what you want to do to them, or what you've been waiting to do to them all day. When they walk through the door, grab them in your arms and say "I've been waiting all day to kiss you all over", that'll take them by surprise. As you start kissing them all over (like you said you would), say things like "You taste so good you have no idea". The dirty talk can even continue after the sex is over by saying "Your tits felt incredible in my mouth just now" or "Your cock felt so hard inside me just now, I loved it!". That should send shivers up their spine.

•   Think About the Timing- Good timing is everything. A single word uttered at the wrong time can quickly kill the arousal you worked so hard to build. As you test the waters, ideally you want to wait until both of you are sufficiently aroused and "hot for each other" before you progress towards the hardcore dirty talk lingo. It's much easier to drop some lustful remarks into the lovemaking session after you're panting and can hardly hold off your lust for each other any longer.

•	Figure Out Their Triggers - Everyone's got a trigger, even if they have never dirty talked before. Trigger words are those special key phrases that turn your partner from a tame lover into a wild stallion. This is where communication once more plays a crucial role as you talk to each other about it. The best way to figure out what your partner's triggers words are is to ask them. Ask and ye shall receive.

•	Try Role-Playing - Sexual fantasies can be extremely arousing. There's nothing like seeing the naughty seen you've tucked away in your mind all this time come to life in front of you. It's like the Disneyland of lovemaking and it's a great excuse to start talking in a way you never have before (i.e. dirty talk). There should be no judgment happening here, respect what your partner's fantasies are. Couples should work together to create an environment where both feel safe enough to reveal their secrets. Maybe your fantasy involves being rescued by a man in uniform as he sweeps you up in his arms and carries you into the bedroom to have his way with you. Maybe in your fantasy, you're the director of an adult movie and you're "directing" your lover about what they need to do onscreen. Tell them how to slowly peel their clothes off in front of the camera, or how to use sex toys to tease their genitals. Your fantasies are only limited by your imagination and if your partner is up for it, anything goes. Role-playing is the perfect opportunity to slip in some dirty lingo, and because you're pretending to be someone else at the time, there's less awkwardness involved.

How to Introduce Your Partner to Dirty Talk

What you like in bed is unique to you. Like your fingerprints, no two people are going to necessarily like the same thing. What kicks your sexual desire into overdrive might be something that makes your partner cringe at the very thought of it. For this endeavor to be a success, couples need to figure out what is going to work for both of them. Desire and pleasure can't be a one-way street in this context. Both partners need to be fully committed to the experience if it is going to work. Admittedly, this can be tricky if you're just getting to know your significant other and you haven't been dating for very long. How do you tell someone you're only starting to get intimate with that you want them to talk dirty to you in bed? That sounds like a disaster waiting to happen. But it doesn't have to be if you play your cards right.

The easiest way to introduce your partner to the hidden pleasure of lustful lingo is to lead by example. Let's say you were with a partner who is not quite as adventurous as you are. They might be taken aback or even shocked if you suddenly come at them full force telling them all the naughty things you would like to do and describing parts of their body using expletives. Introduce your partner to it by starting slow with less forceful language to start. Watch the way they react and respond to your verbal cues and any physical cues that might accompany your words. When it comes to dirty talk, not everyone wants the same delivery. Some couples may be into the sweet, kinky, or romantic kind of dirty talk. Others are turned on by anything that relates to their fantasies. It does not have to be raunchy or hardcore all the time, it depends entirely on the couple and what works best.

How do you work up to it though, and casually bring it up in conversation without pushing against your partner's boundaries too much? Well, opportunity knocks in different ways, one of which would be when you're watching a movie together as an example of one such scenario. Wait for the opportune moment, and during a particularly steamy scene on screen, casually say "I think it's incredibly sexy the way they used dirty talk there, what do you think?". Another way to ease this topic into the conversation is when you're kissing and cuddling each other. As your kisses intensify, whisper in their ear between kisses what they would like to hear in bed. Ask them to tell you what turns them on. In return, tell them what does it for you and what you would like to hear them say. Sexual desires and fantasies are perfectly normal and nothing to be ashamed about. You've got your secret fantasies and you can bet that your partner has them too.

What happens if your partner is still not a fan of dirty talk despite your best efforts? That's okay, the important thing is that you don't stress too much over this until it creates tension between you. It can be frustrating and disappointing to find out that you're not on the same page, but there is always a solution to every conundrum. The solution in this case? Try to find a compromise. Talk to each other and work out what a happy medium could be so you still get the dirty talking you've been craving but without making your partner too uncomfortable at the same time. If your partner is not keen on using profanities, work out a system where you whisper compliments to each other instead. Or you could ask if they would consider being more vocal in bed, not with their words, but with the sounds they make. A few well-placed "mmms" and "aahhhs" could still get the job done.

If after all of that your partner still gives you a firm NO in the dirty talk department, it is important that you respect their wishes. No one should feel forced into doing something they don't want to do, especially when it comes to sex. Let them know you respect their point of view and you understand where they're coming from, and then explain where you are coming from and why this matters to you. Help them understand what dirty talk means to you in a way that they can relate to. If they don't feel forced into it, they might be more willing to listen and consider the possibility if they know that it is going to make you happy. Ultimately, everyone has a right to say no to what they don't feel comfortable doing in bed. Talk about it, but don't resent your significant other if the answer is not what you want to hear. Remember you wouldn't want to feel pressured or forced into doing something you don't want to do to either.

Does Erotic Questioning Help?

It is certainly one way a couple could ease erotic talk into their regular bedroom routine. This method works like an ice breaker, which is one reason why it is effective, particularly for couples who feel shy around each other as they try to dirty up their words for the first time. Asking your partner these questions lets you gauge what their preferences are, or even what they secretly desire that they were too nervous or shy to share with you prior to this.

For this approach to work, let your emotions and desires flow freely when you're kissing and holding your partner. Slowly run your fingers over his or her body. Stroke the back of their neck just behind the ear before sliding your fingers around the front as you work your way down to their chest. As you alternate the areas you touch your partner, ask them what feels good. Which spot made them gasp a little more when your fingers fluttered over the area? Say "Does that feel good when I touch you there?".

Examples for the Beginner In You

It never hurts to be prepared with a few phrases up your sleeve to test the waters with and see which ones you respond to best as a couple. Ease into the process by using some of the following phrases as a guide:

•	You have no idea what I want to do you right now

•	God, baby, you taste so damn good you're turning me on

•	Oh yes, right there, that feels so good. Don't stop touching my _______ oh that feels so good

•	More, more, don't stop oh I want more

- That thing you do with your tongue drives me crazy

- I'm so hard for you right now I'm going to f**k you until you beg me to stop

- Don't wear any underwear under your skirt today. It's giving me ideas

- It drives me crazy when you're moaning my name

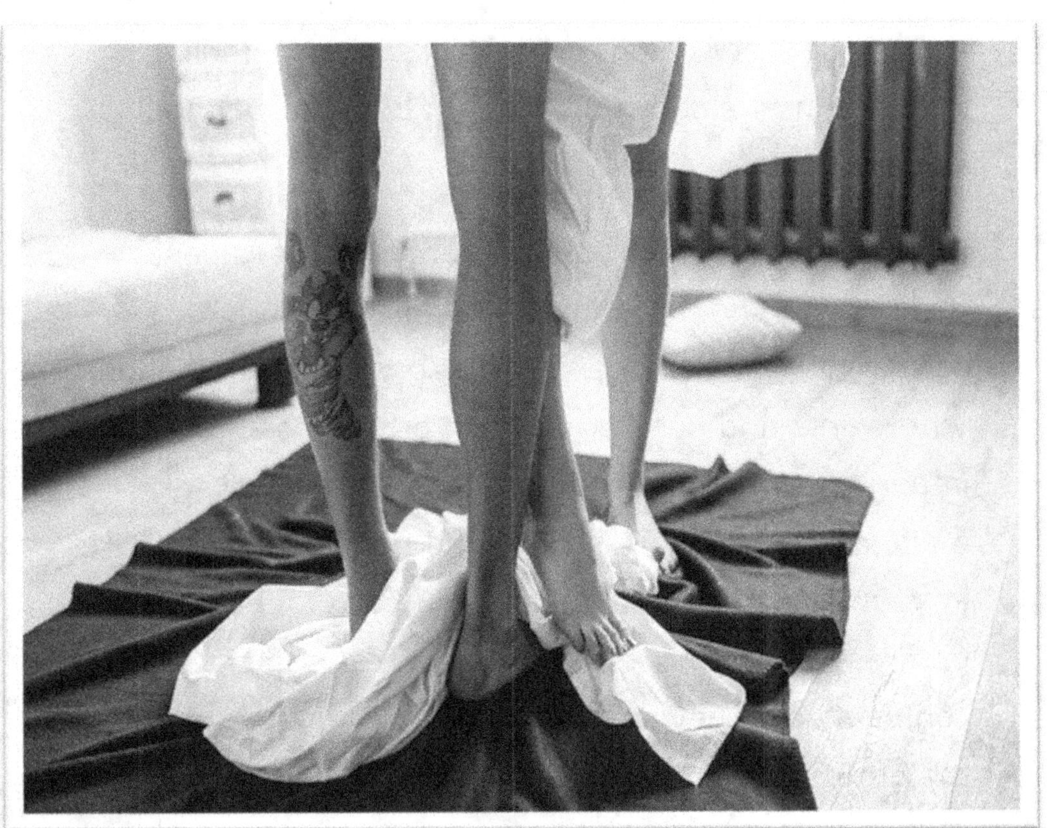

Chapter 3 The Benefits of Dirty Talk

Communication is the secret to accomplishment in a relationship, but it is particularly important in sexual relationships. For a certain something, it's been scientifically demonstrated to expand satisfaction on both sides of the equation—various studies, including a recent investigation from the analysts at Temple University, have discovered that transparently communicating about sexual needs and health has all the earmarks of being a strong predictor of feeling satisfied in a relationship, both in bed and when all is said in done.

But the estimation of verbal intercourse goes past, making you two more joyful. Important though satisfaction is in any sexual relationship, talking about your wants and needs with each other has other important emotional benefits. It brings you closer, making you feel more secure and progressively secure in your relationship. It causes you both to feel progressively competent and, as a result, increasingly confident. You never again need to think about what the other individual wants and marvel whether or not you're doing it right—and neither of you needs to "counterfeit it" and pretend to appreciate something rather than supporting apprehension that you will be scorned or hurt the other individual's emotions.

It's likewise vital, both for the health of your relationship and your very own prosperity, to have the option to talk about physical concerns, including scatters, disabilities, or other restorative worries that may affect your sexual function. It's much better to bring such issues up as quickly as time permits to guarantee both your safety and your partner's. Regardless of whether neither of you currently has a particular medicinal or physical issue to consider, essentially having the option to communicate what feels better and what doesn't can go far towards preventing sex-related wounds and infections.

Being in agreement in terms of play styles and toys is important for emotional and physical health, too. If one of you is into increasingly in-your-face exotic play including beating and leather whips while the other doesn't care to get more adventurous than trying on a soft satin blindfold on occasion, your solution ought not be to "suck it up" and pretend to make the most of your partner's wrinkles—nor should you try and power your partner to be into yours. Communication means being available to each other's interests and needs and discovering solutions to sexual problems that will help you both feel increasingly satisfied, all through the bedroom.

Step by step instructions to Communicate Effectively

Obviously, communication isn't just an issue of opening your mouth and talking. So as to have any effect, you need to realize how to articulate your sentiments unmistakably and affectionately—and how to listen and react to your partner's wants with attentiveness and compassion.

Introducing the Topic

The first stage in figuring out how to communicate effectively is making sense of how to start a conversation in the first spot. Realize that the timing may never be perfect—and trying to wait until it is may keep you procrastinating long past the perfect fateful opening. That being stated, trying to suggest a tricky bedroom topic during an unimaginably inopportune moment can be just as terrible.

• Don't start the conversation in an as of now emotionally-charged discourse. In particular, trying to talk about a sensitive subject during a fight will undoubtedly leave an awful taste in both of your mouths, and once in a while (if at any point) results in an actual resolution.

• Do be available to communicate your needs in the bedroom—while you're sleeping. It's true that progressively genuine; in-depth conversations ought to presumably take place somewhere else—in case you're thinking of trying BDSM just because, for instance, it's important to talk about preferences and limits well early. But for increasingly straightforward or off the cuff requests, while you're together in bed may actually be the best spot to bring them up. Talking about sex can be sexy; don't stress over destroying the state of mind by requesting something different or new!

• Don't use sexy time as an excuse to manipulate your partner emotionally. It's alright to request what you want—it's not alright to try and extortion or force them into accomplishing something they unmistakably would prefer not to do.

• Do take the initiative. Your partner can't guess what you might be thinking anything else than you can peruse theirs. Don't expect them to realize something is up instinctively; it's dependent upon you to represent yourself.

If you need help getting started, think about utilizing an online study on sexual inclinations to break the ice.

Talking to Your Partner

• Keep quiet and stay positive. Rather than basically criticizing your partner's tastes or technique, outline your requests in a positive light at whatever point conceivable. For instance, in the event that they insist on similar old positions without fail, but you'd like to try utilizing a rooster ring or another couples' vibrator to zest things up, don't chastise them for being exhausting or traditional. Instead, tell them how you think another toy could be a reviving difference in pace.

• Don't let disgrace or dread of vulnerability keep you quiet. Don't be challenging for yourself in case you're not into utilizing toys for areola play like your partner is or you have A, dull, secret crimp you don't think they'll share. You may not generally concur on what's hot and so forth, but that's not so important as having the option to talk about these distinctions and find sexy solutions that work for you both. This is doubly true on the off chance that you've got a significant issue that should be tended to; the more you wait to bring it up, mainly if it's a medicinal concern, the more regrettable it will get. Keep in mind, maintaining your health and prosperity ought to consistently take priority over staying away from unbalanced conversations or trying not to ruin the moment.

• Try not to overpower your partner. Making some noise isn't equivalent to talking over your partner, and communicating doesn't mean blurting out everything that's at the forefront of your thoughts at the same time. Try to tackle just each issue in turn, and on the off chance that you've got a significantly extreme request as a primary concern, consider working up to it steadily. In case you're into S&M, and your partner is timid or saved, for instance, you most likely won't end up hopping into the deep end. Be eager to go moderate and take things slowly and carefully, and be happy to stop if and when your partner asks you to, not just when you feel like it.

Listening to Your Partner

Just like your relationship, your conversations ought to be a two-way street. Make sure to let your partner realize you esteem their thoughts and sentiments as much as you want them to respect yours by remembering these three tips:

• Listen actively and respectfully. Regardless of how enormous or how little their requests, it's essential to let your partner realize that you're present in the conversation and ready not just to listen but to think about what they are stating, whether that implies acting on their request or finding a mutually pleasant alternative. It's similarly critical to ensure you don't disgrace them for shouting out, regardless of whether you don't understand or concur with their inclinations—otherwise, they'll be significantly less prone to open up to you again in the future.

• Ask thoughtful questions. The secret to excellent communication isn't gesturing and concurring; it's creation certain you're both in agreement. The best method to do this is to ask your partner inquiries that assist them with making some noise or explain what they've just said.

• Be available to suggestions, but clear on your limits. Be that as it may, know your hard limits—things you absolutely cannot, or won't, try under any circumstances—and express them obviously and transparently with your partner—before things get hot and substantial.

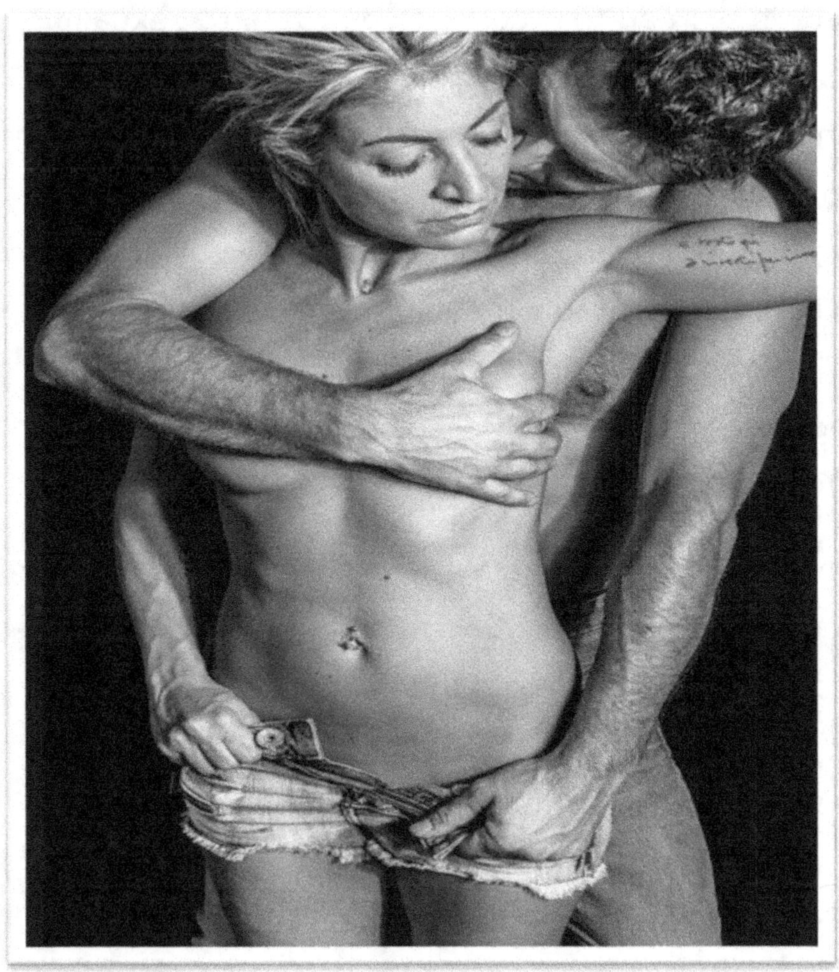

Chapter 4 Increase your sexual vocabulary

Our Early Lessons in Sex and Communication

Most small kids are vigorously protected from conversations about sex. It's viewed as incredibly taboo for youngsters to hear or see anything sexual. There is a dread that early introduction to sexuality will corrupt, confuse, or traumatize little youngsters. Many individuals have had the experience of strolling into a room and having adults quiet immediately. Sometimes we can tell just enough of what they are talking about to know the subject. This can create a feeling of amazement, mystery, or disgrace that progresses toward becoming associated with sex.

As individuals become more established, the conversation tends to stay taboo. Individuals become effectively embarrassed because they don't have any great models or how to talk about sex. Their entire life, they've been indicated that it's taboo and embarrassing. These sentiments can be exacerbated by an absence of appropriate sex education. Not just have individuals demonstrated that it's uncomfortable, but there can be a gigantic hole in understanding.

Awful (Or No) Communication Leads to Bad Sex

It's a pretty basic fantasy that our partners should have the option to guess our thoughts and recognize what we want. A few people don't think of it as sexy to need to inquire. Others feel that it will ruin the state of mind. The truth is that neither of these things is true. A few people discover talking about what they're doing or going to do, unfathomably sexy. It's often alluded to as dirty talk.

But what occurs if we go with the silent methodology?

Lots of things can emerge when individuals neglect to communicate. For starters, consent may not be obtained, or on the off chance that it is, limits might be crossed. Two individuals might not have the exact thought of what sex implies. One individual may consider butt-centric sex reasonable game while the other was thinking oral or vaginal. What if one individual thinks an aspect of BDSM as a regular part of sex? Talking can create clear limits.

Another regular thing that can happen when there's an inability to communicate is phony climaxes. Sometimes individuals feel a lot of strain to satisfy their partner. This can go both ways. The individual who is playing out a sex act on their partner is trying typically trying hard to convince them. The individual getting that attention may likewise feel constrained to give their partner satisfying information that they are working admirably. If the individual isn't comfortable communicating what they want, they may counterfeit pleasure to move the activities along. Faking the climax not just betrays the trust of the partner, but it additionally expands the opportunity they will return to similar moves because they were persuaded it's what their partner wanted.

We end up with individuals losing interest and satisfaction in sex. Couples wind up having less sex while it builds the dissatisfaction of their time together.

Communication in Sex Increases Our Sexual Pleasure

At the point when we articulate what we want unmistakably, our partner gets the opportunity to choose if they can and want to meet our needs. It's a simple step to having all the more satisfying and pleasurable sex. We are likewise teaching our partners to be better lovers for us. Much of the time, it can be as straightforward as letting them know to stay focused on or move away from a particular spot, accelerate or delayed down, or hit us with some dirty talk.

Being open about communicating our sexual wants can open up some other entryways also. There is an entire domain of sexual experience and sensations that individuals may wish to investigate but isn't an automatic default for most individuals. At the point when we can talk straightforwardly with our partner, we can talk about studying a portion of those wants. It allows couples to try some different things and investigate their sexual fantasies. Not just will this lead to all the more satisfying sex, but it can likewise develop the obligations of intimacy in the relationship.

Practice Makes Perfect When Talking About Sex

In case you're not used to talking about your sexual want, it can feel cumbersome when you first start doing it. The trick is to keep the conversation occurring with your partner. Be supportive of one another and keep the conversation as light as would be prudent. This will help urge you to talk about it more. Practice makes perfect.

It's easy to talk dirty, but it becomes even easier as soon as you understand how to pick your sexual vocabulary. What many people don't realize is that your sexual vocabulary also speaks volumes about your relationship.

Ready to learn a little more about sexual vocabulary and phrases that are going to create a dirty talking atmosphere with your partner that is purely and simply orgasmic? It's what sexual vocabulary is all about, and once you develop your own go-to phrases and words, you'll feel that much more comfortable talking dirty to your man.

What Your Vocabulary Says:

Unless you're using clinical terms like scrotum and penetration with your partner (please, please don't do that), you already have a bit of your sexual vocabulary hanging out in your head, making the process that much easier.

There are five types of sexual vocabulary that you may or may not be using, and you can choose to use whichever one makes you comfortable and gets your partner aroused. Personally, I would avoid the first one at all cost. Most people find that using clinical terms can be even more awkward than if you're trying to use slang you're unaccustomed to. Remember to keep your tone relaxed, and you will start to gravitate towards whichever one you feel more comfortable with. Don't be afraid to push your comfort level. You'll never know where to draw the line if you don't step over it at least once.

Clinical Terms:

Clinical terms just aren't sexy, and when you say that you'd like to be penetrated, it's not the same as asking him to make love to you or straight out fuck you. Some terms that would probably make him go limp as a noodle include fellatio, scrotum, anal penetration, cunnilingus, and copulate. The idea of copulating is not the same as the idea of making love, screwing, or fucking like animals until you both collapse on the bed fully satisfied with each other. Let's just pinky promise to avoid clinical terms altogether when we're trying to sound sexy or talk dirty.

Standard Erotic Language:

This is the type of vocabulary that you'd find in an erotic novel, and it includes ejaculate, erection, and climax. This may be great for you, but most men want something that is a little cruder. However, if you're just getting into talking dirty, this may be easier at first. You can use it as a stepping stone to getting a little more comfortable with actually talking dirty. Baby steps are better than no steps.

Oral Sex Slang:

This is sort of a category all on its own, and that's because it's a category of sex all on its own that is performed often. There is nothing wrong with oral sex, and chances are you've either done it to him or he's done it to you. Some slang terms include going down, giving head, clit, and even boner. A blowjob is not actually an oral sex slang term, and instead it falls under crude language. Talking dirty right before he goes down on you or vice versa is one way to start, as it's not too crude, but it's still specific enough to make him aroused, especially if you add a sexy voice.

Everyday Sexual Vocabulary:

There are terms that we use every day, and these are the terms that you are more likely to use with your friends if you're chatting about sexual experiences. These terms include penis, boobs, making love, nipples, and pussy. These are all okay to say, and you need to get comfortable with saying them if you want to talk dirty successfully.

Crude Sexual Language:

Thinking a lady would never talk like this? You're probably right. But guess what, we leave our prim and proper lady shoes at the bedroom door where they belong. I know you've heard the saying about a man wanting a lady in the streets but a freak in the bed. Well, it's true. Not just something guys say. Newsflash! They actually mean it! Don't believe me? Got a good guy friend? Ask him. There's just something about those bad girls that has them thinking about it all day long.

If you want rough, dirty, exhausting sex, you will probably eventually gravitate more towards adding verbs to naughty crude language, such as blowjob, tits, balls, pussy, cunt, cock, screw, and fuck. Of course, some of them you may be shouting, but try to form coherent sentences with these to talk dirty before you are pushed over the edge of the cliff and into orgasm with your very open and happy sexual partner.

Hint: This is most men's favorite playground. By far.

What It Says About Your Relationship:

With women, no matter which one you're using, you'll probably feel closer to your partner.

If a man is using clinical terms with you, he's probably not comfortable with you at all. Now that I think about it, he may not even be comfortable with sex! He's probably not as comfortable if he's using erotic terms as well, and he may feel like he's having to try too hard. It's more natural to use every day sexual language as well as crude language. Oral sex language comes all on its own, but the comfort levels between both of you should be as high as they can. This will lead to a better relationship as well as better sex, so don't feel like you have to hold back.

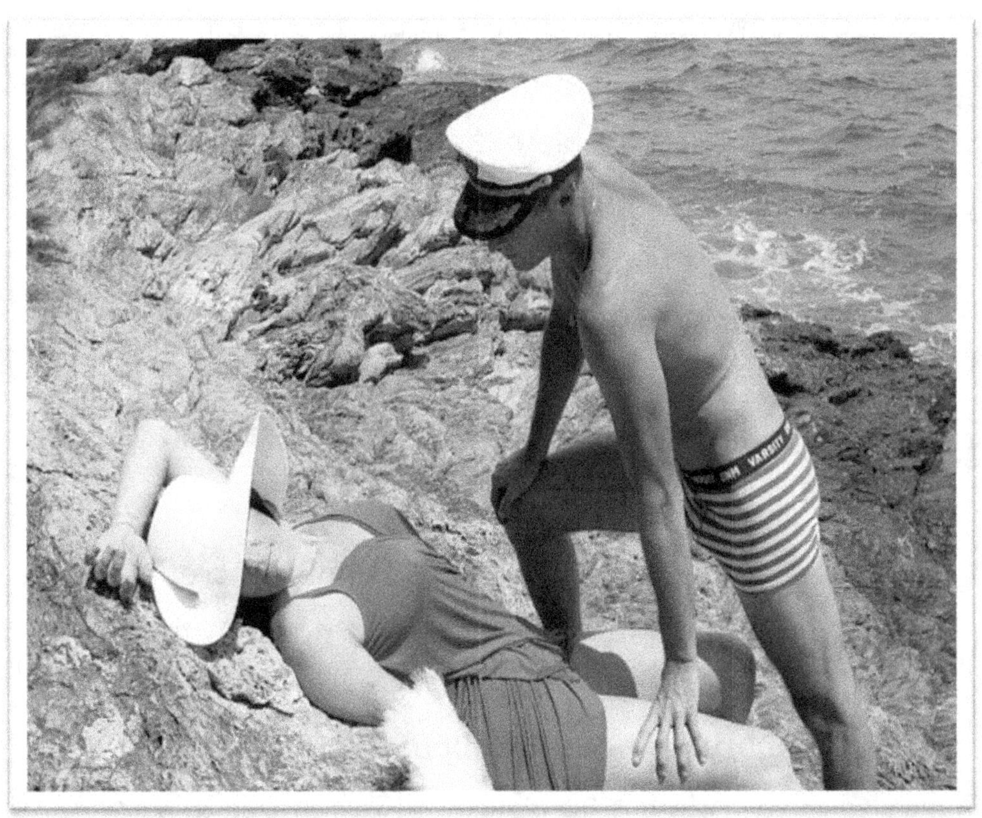

Chapter 5 Dirty Talk Phrases To Get You Started

Let's get down to business. If you have been wondering exactly what dirty things to say to your partner, you'll get ample examples in this chapter. While these lines can have a great positive impact on your partner and overall sex life, it is better to customize them to suit your particular situation. Your partner can tell if you are just recanting things you read off a book because it won't sound real and it won't be tailored to him or her.

You can use these examples as a guide for creating your own original lines. Talking dirty doesn't mean blabbing away throughout sex. A few simple but well-timed naughty remarks are all that is required to take your sex experience up a notch. Remember to vary your lines so they won't become boring. The best way to do that is to tune into the sensations you feel, the sexual desires you want to be fulfilled, and then vocalize them.

If you find it too awkward to be verbally expressive, tell yourself that you are temporarily switching into a different role to test whether or not dirty talks are for you. Now, let loose, get into the moment, and flow with it.

Since not everyone is on the same level of openness and comfortability, I have grouped the examples into three different levels:

- **Beginner level**: This is for those who want to give dirty talk a trial or for those testing the waters with a new partner. The language here is easy, suggestive, and can be considered safe even for highly modest people.

- **Intermediary level**: This is for those who want to improve their naughty bedroom language. The phrases in this section are raunchier and can get your man harder or woman wetter. If you are new to being naughty, you may find these examples a bit too challenging.

- **Advanced level**: The examples here are for those who have no qualms sharing their deepest fantasies with their partner and are better used when you are very sure your partner is on the same page as you with regards to dirty talks. The phrases here are extremely explicit and not meant for the faint-hearted.

You will also find suggested phrases that can be used before sex (to build sexual tension), after sex (to maintain sexual momentum) and even dirty things to say in public places. I suggest that you sift through these pre and post-sex dirty talks and select the ones that you are most comfortable with. Remember to do a preliminary check with your partner before using these phrases even if you are intimate with them. It is safer to be sure than to assume.

Beginner Level

For ladies (what your man wants to hear)

During sex

The following phrases are best tailored for women to use during sex. Some of these lines can also be used during foreplay. Ladies, your man would love to hear you say these words:

1. That feels so amazing!

2.God! That's feels so good.

3.I'm so wet right now.

4.I'm dripping wet for you!

5.I love it when you whisper those words in my ears.

6.I love it when you do that to me.

7.I love it when you caress me like that.

8.I love the feel of your strong arms around me.

9.I feel so sexy just staying here in your arms.

10.I love it when you eat me up.

11. It feels good when you are inside me.

12.You look so handsome/manly, my love.

13.You have the body of a sex god!

14.Lie back, relax, and let me take good care of you.

15. I need to hold you tight right now.

16.I'm going to kiss you so softly you'll lose your mind!

17. Relax, let me warm you up.

18. Baby, come closer and set my flesh/soul on fire.

19. Make me come, baby.

20. I can't wait to have your arms wrapped around me.

21. Kiss my lips, darling.

22. I want to feel your warm breath on my face.

23. Come take my breath away.

24. Put your hands between my thighs.

25. Come tell me all about those dirty little secrets.

26. I want to feel your weight on top of me.

27. Come taste me.

28. I want to feel you deep inside of me.

29. Take me.

30. Choke me!

31. Ride me.

32. Faster.

33. Deeper.

34.Harder.

35.Hit it harder.

36.Right there.

37.That's the spot!

38.Let's do this all night.

39.Slowly, my love, slowly.

40.Tear me up!

41.Pull my hair, please.

42.Spank me!

43.Fill me up, please!

44.I can't take this suspense any longer. Come take me, darling!

45.Squeeze me tight.

46.Run those manly hands all over my body.

47.Keep going, don't stop!

48.Tell me how you want it.

49.What dirty thing do you have in mind?

50.How would you like to be served?

51. What naughty things would you like me to do to you?

52.Hold me tight and never let go.

53.Undress me, baby, and do to me as you please.

54.Take me and do to me whatever you please, my love.

55.I can tell you want me.

56.Tell me your secret fantasies.

57.Come practice what you preach.

58.I'm all yours, baby. All yours.

59.Show me all the naughty things you can do.

60.Show me how much you want me.

61.I love your warm breath between my thighs.

62.Kiss me gently on my lips, boobs, and between my thighs.

63.Come for me baby, come so hard.

64.Have your way with me tonight.

65.You own me, my love.

66.You whisper in my ears and make me weak in my knees.

67.Dominate me and make me beg.

68.Strip me naked with those sexy eyes.

69.The look in your eyes gives me the shivers.

70.Your wish is my command.

71. I need you so bad right now.

72.Tonight, I'm doing all the work while you lay back and enjoy my touch.

73.Touch me like no one has ever touched me before.

74.Touch my lips. No, not with your hands but with your sexy lips.

75.You kiss my lips and I can't seem to think straight anymore.

76.Take me right now! I want to melt into you!

For men (what your woman wants to hear)

During sex

The following phrases are best suited for men during sex. You can use some of these lines during foreplay too. Men, don't be a painful bore during sex. Your woman would love to hear you say these words:

1. You're making me hard as a rock.

2.Come here darling, sit on my lap.

3.Say my name.

4.Who's your daddy?

5.I like the sexy look in your eyes.

6.Come here, you hot, sexy goddess.

7.The look in your eyes is making me hard.

8.I want to kiss those sexy lips of yours.

9.You look like an angel when you kiss my lip.

10.Your hair smells like heaven to me.

11. You look so ravishing right now I feel like devouring you!

12. Keep stroking me like that, baby.

13. I like it when you use your tongue.

14. Right there, baby.

15. Say it again, slowly.

16. I love it when you take charge.

17. Tonight, you are in control.

18. You're so hot!

19. You have the most gorgeous body ever.

20. Tease me, baby, until I lose control.

21. You taste so sweet, baby.

22. You are so wet.

23. You're warm, wet, and slippery!

24. You are so tight.

25. I want to taste you.

26. You're so good with your tongue.

27. You have magic fingers.

28. Grind on me slowly.

29.Spread your legs for me.

30.Are you ready for me?

31.Do you like it when I do that?

32.Daddy's coming for you, baby.

33.I want to ride you slowly.

34.Get ready for the ride of your life!

35.Are you feeling this?

36.Say it like you mean it.

37.You're wild like a tigress, and it turns me on.

38.I'm almost there.

39.Lay back let me slowly kiss every inch of your sexy body.

40.I'm going to make you scream my name.

41.I want to rip off your clothes and do to you all the naughty things I've been thinking about all day long.

42.Your sexy body is turning me on.

43.You're so delicious my love.

44.Your body is so perfect.

45.Tonight, you belong to me.

46.I know you want me inside you, filling and tearing you up, don't you?

47.I've waited for your sexy body all day. Come here let me show you what I have in mind.

48.I'm going to kiss you anywhere you choose. Show me where you want my lips.

49.Your lips are so warm and soft.

50.I'm so hard just by looking at your sexy body.

51. Place your hand on my chest and feel what my heart is saying.

52.You are my naughty girl.

53.I'll take it easy and slow, and then flip you over and give it to you rough and fast.

54.You're just too delicious I wish I could eat you all day.

55.I get harder when you moan with pleasure.

56.I'll run my hands through your hair and nibble on your ears while I stick it from behind.

57.I like the feel of your soft skin. It sets my groin on fire!

58.Tonight, all your sexual fantasies are about to be fulfilled by this sex god.

59.Just the sight of you turns me on.

60.Come closer baby let me run my fingers down your spine.

61.Get on your knees and beg for it.

62.It feels so good when you stroke me that way.

63.You make me long helplessly for your body.

64.You bring out the wild animal in me.

65.I can never get tired of making love to you.

66.Your soft, sweet boobs against my chest... mmm... this is pure heaven!

Intermediate

For ladies (what your man wants to hear)

During sex

These phrases target your man's ego, decrease your inhibition of filthy words, and increase your boldness to express your intimate desires and sexual fantasies.

1. Your cock/dick is perfect for me. I love it like crazy.

2.Drive me wild with that big, strong dick of yours.

3.Relax and let me make you cum like never before.

4.The gods must envy your dick. It's a sight to behold!

5.Make that dick throb for me, baby.

6.I totally adore your gorgeous dick/cock.

7.I'm madly in love with your dick.

8.I worship this gorgeous cock you have dangling before my eyes.

9.I love how your cock pulsates inside me.

10.I'm addicted to your cock.

11. The size of the bulge in your pants tells me you're ready to fuck me.

12.You're good with your tongue.

13.I love your wet tongue on my hard nipples.

14.Lick me again, slowly this time.

15. Cup my boobs and squeeze them.

16.I fucking love how you ride me.

17. You drive me crazy when you kiss my pussy lips.

18.I love sucking you until you cum.

19.Pound me hard.

20.Tonight I'm your prisoner. Punish me with that big cock of yours.

21.I like the look on your face when you cum for me.

22.Fuck me in front of the mirror, my love.

23.Look into my eyes when you cum.

24.Tell me how good it feels when you fuck me.

25.Go in deep! Fucking make me pregnant.

26.I like the feel of your hard cock in my mouth.

27.How do you like my sexy little ass?

28.I love it when you nibble on my hard nipples.

29.You deserve an award for fucking me this good.

30.Bang me from behind.

31.Jerk off for me, please.

32.I made the bed already, but I don't mind messing up the sheets with you.

33.I want to feel the bulge in your pants against my ass.

34.Shove that monstrous dick in my pussy... every inch of it.

35.Tell me every naughty detail of what you want to do to me.

36.I am your sex slave. I'll do anything for your cum.

37.Fuck me again, please.

38.I love it when you grab my butt-cheek that way.

39. Tonight, let me be your naughty little girl.

40. This pussy needs you deep inside right now.

41. Your cock redefines sex.

42. Lay that macho body on me.

43. Where did you keep this cock all of my life?

44. Yes, I like being your dirty little girl.

45. Bury your cute boyish face in mommy's voluptuous boobs.

46. Get on your knees and kiss my ass, now!

47. Kiss my lips... no, my lips down there!

48. Go in deeper, deeper!

49. I love how you growl when you are about to cum.

50. Give me a warm pussy massage, please.

51. Give me a full-body massage... and full-body orgasm.

52. I want those nice-looking fingers inside me.

53. Your cock tastes and feels good in my mouth.

54.Shove it in, baby, shove it!

55.Bite me all over.

56.I like how you slide your hard cock in and out of my wet pussy.

57.This pussy is dripping wet for you.

58.Flip me over and ride me in my favorite position.

59.I love the way your cock feels in my tight hole.

60.Spread my ass cheek and shove that big cock in my tight little pussy.

61.Fucking you is heavenly!

62.I want you to fuck me silly!

63.Your hard cock rocks my world!

64.I like lollipops, but not as much as your sweet dick.

65.I want to suck on your dick all night.

66.The thought of your hard cock sliding into my tight pussy leaves me shaking like a leaf.

For men (what your woman wants to hear)

During sex

Your woman will feel more wanted, needed, loved, and appreciated when you say these words.

1. I love it when you squeeze my dick with your cunt/pussy.

2. Your touch makes my dick/cock so hard it hurts a little.

3. I love how you suck my hard cock.

4. You sure know how to use your tongue to make me go wild.

5. Holy shit! I'm going to explode if you keep doing that!

6. Your ass looks so perfect from this angle.

7. My little good girl, suck on daddy's cock.

8. Come let me play with your tight little pussy.

9. I want to eat dessert off your sexy body.

10. I love the feeling of sheer ecstasy I get when you ride my cock.

11. I want to see how soaking wet you are.

12. Your warm pussy makes me want to spend all night inside you.

13. I want to explode inside of you!

14. Bring those beautiful breasts of yours here! I want to suck them so bad!

15. I want to bury my face between your thighs.

16. I'll circle my tongue around your clit until you quiver from sheer pleasure.

17. I am entranced by the sight of your wet cunt.

18. Your vagina got me intoxicated.

19. Sit on this dick and ride me like a pony.

20. Tilt your ass up a bit let me get a good view of your honey pot.

21. Your pussy grows sweeter by the day. I can't wait to taste it again.

22. How do you want me to fuck you, slow or fast?

23. I love how you grab the sheets when I push my dick all the way.

24.You're so fucking wet.

25.Turn around and bless me with the sight of your perfect ass.

26.My balls are lonely and cold. Would you warm them up with your mouth, please?

27.I love the sound you make when my tongue is between your legs.

28.Clench that sweet pussy around my cock.

29.I'm dying to have a cock massage.

30.I like the feel of your soft hands. They should be holding my hard cock.

31.Spread it just like that... yeah.

32.Tonight, I want you to wear only this when I ride you from behind.

33.I love how your tits dangle when I take you from behind.

34.I'll make those boobs clap so hard until you call me your daddy.

35.Bend over let me oil up your hot ass.

36.Make that ass clap for daddy.

37.I like the feel of your hands when you shave my dick and balls.

38.Dig those nails into my ass cheek when I'm about to cum hard inside you.

Advance Level

For ladies (what your man wants to hear)

During sex

These phrases are for you if your man doesn't mind getting extra filthy and naughty. Some of these phrases sound demeaning, but they are not meant to debase the female gender. I strongly suggest that you use them only in the context of a loving relationship. A lady who uses these dirty phrases for men she meets casually runs the risk of being considered irresponsible. Be reckless all you want, but let it be with a man who still holds you in high regard after all the dirty talk.

1. Shove every inch of that cock into my wet cunt.

2.Call me your dirty whore/slut.

3.Fuck me, baby. Fuck me like your life depends on it!

4.Tear up that pussy!

5.You own this fucking pussy!

6.Fuck this pussy like you own it.

7.Eat this pussy like you mean it.

8.Your cum tastes so delicious.

9.Cum in my mouth, please. I want to taste your cum.

10.I want to suck your cock until you shoot your load.

11. Lick my wet little pussy.

12.Cum hard for me, daddy.

13.Cum inside me, darling.

14.Cum all over me, my love.

15. Fuck my pretty face, darling.

16.I'm your little slut/whore.

17. Suck my clit, baby.

18.Let me be your sex slut tonight.

19.Oh, fucking shit! I'm coming!

20.I love the taste of my cum on your fucking cock.

21.You fuck like a god!

22.I want you to shoot your load all over my face!

23.Thank you for pounding me so hard.

24.I'm hungry for your hard cock right now.

25.Watch how my tits jiggle as I ride your hard cock.

26.This pussy is meant for your dick.

27.Fuck me like a dog!

28.Play with my wet cunt while I jerk off your hard cock.

29.Suck on my tits while I ride you like crazy.

30.Tease my clit with the tip of your dick.

31.Please master let me give you a blow job.

32.I'll do anything you say because I'm your little bitch.

33.Do to me all the kinky things you've been thinking about.

34.I'm bending over for you. How do you like the view?

35.Spank this ass and fuck my brains out!

36.Push me against the wall and fuck my pussy till it hurts.

37.I love it when you flick your tongue against my clit.

38.Fuck me as if you are closing a multimillion-dollar deal!

39.I'm going to squeeze your cock so tight that you'll explode inside of me.

40.Come dick me down with your monster cock.

41.I can feel your thick cum inside me.

42.Tell me I'm your dirtiest slut ever.

43.Put that cock back in my wet warm hole and stop whining like a little wimp!

44.I'm going to sit on your fucking face until you make me cum.

45.Come on! Tongue-fuck this pussy!

46. Do you fucking own this your pussy or what?

47. You've been a bad boy! It's time for your punishment.

48. I love it when you masturbate and cum hard for me.

49. Pull my hair when you shoot your load.

50. I love it when you lick the creamy candy off my pussy.

51. If you shave my hairy pussy, I'll suck your cock until you beg me to stop.

52. Eat my cunt until I beg you to stop.

53. Make me scream your name.

54. Lay me on this desk and fuck me like your secretary.

55. Lick my tight asshole.

For men (what your woman wants to hear)

During sex

Not every woman will like to hear these phrases, so be sure about the lady in question before using these lines for her. Consider these filthy talks as tools to heighten the sexual enjoyment for both of you, and not in any way a description of the woman you are with.

1. I love it when you tease the tip of my cock with your tongue.

2.Beg me, you little bitch.

3.You've been a good girl all day. It's time to reward your tight little pussy.

4.Say my fucking name when you cum, bitch.

5.Get undressed and lie down. I'm about to fuck you mercilessly.

6.I'll fuck you until your whole body is shaking.

7.Go on all fours and beg me to cum.

8.Get on your knees and swallow this cum.

9.Cum hard for me, baby.

10.Rub your pussy for me.

11. Suck this fucking cock like a pro.

12.Make me cum with no hands baby, just your slutty mouth.

13.Touch yourself, I want to see you make yourself cum.

14.I'll pound you so hard you'll forget your name.

15. Gag on my hard cock.

16.I want you to lick your cum off my cock.

17. Sit on my face let me breathe in the sweet smell of your wet cunt.

18.Get on your knees and suck me till I cum.

19.Stroke me faster. I want to cum in your hands.

20.I feel like sticking my cock in all your holes.

21.Lick my balls like a dirty little slut.

22.Drench me in your pussy juice.

23.I'm going to drench you in my warm cum tonight.

24. Lick my balls, you bitch!

25. Bend over, you naughty little girl. You deserve some spanking.

26. Give me that amazing blow job while I eat your pussy in a 69 position.

27. I'll choke you with my hard cock until you gasp for breath!

28. Choke on it, you dirty little whore.

29. Your fucking ass looks so hot when you bend over.

30. Stretch that pussy for daddy, come on, do it!

Pre-Sex Dirty Talks

The following phrases are best used to build sexual tension long before sex. Consider them verbal foreplay that keeps your partner in the mood for sex all day.

1. I can't wait to put my hands all over you tonight.

2. You're going to need all your strength for tonight, so start saving it.

3. I'm going to show you my a few new tricks tonight.

4.I want you to suck on my tits now so I'll such on your cock later.

5.I see that huge bulge in your pants. I can't wait to put my mouth over it.

6.Guess what? I'm soaking wet for you right now. Would you like to dive in and explore?

7.Tonight, I'll give it to you from behind.

8.Tonight. On the counter. I'll bend you over.

9.Why haven't we had sex in the kitchen? Let's try that when you get back.

10.Let's do something kinky tonight. Any ideas?

Post-Sex Dirty Talk

The following phrases are best used after sex. It could be immediately after sex or even a couple of days after.

1. I can't seem to get last night off my mind. You were so amazing!

2.You sure know how to use that tongue of yours. I still shiver when I think of what you did to my clit.

3.Get off my thoughts already! I can't concentrate. All I see is your cock.

4.Even after all these days, my sheets still smell of you.

5.It is funny how I like all the dirty names you called me last night.

6.Thinking about how hard you came last time is getting me horny.

7.I can't wait to get you over here again.

8.You won last night. I demand a rematch.

9.The way you moan and groan with pleasure last time makes me want to have you again, tonight.

10.Thank you for breaking me out of my conservative shell. I look forward to learning more dirty tricks from you, my naughty teacher.

11. You made me giggle like an innocent virgin last night with the way you kept whispering those naughty things in my ears.

12.You definitely know how to ride a cock! That was an amazing experience. I can't wait to spend another quality time with you next weekend.

13.I'mgonna christen you Priapus, the sexy god! Last night, that cock of yours brought out the bitch in me!

14.You shaved me clean and licked me clean! Thank you.

15. No one ever sucked me the way you did last night. You're awesome!

Dirty Compliments That Can Lead to Sex

Use these lines when you want to get your partner to want sex by giving them sexy complementing.

1. Your lips are so moist I feel like kissing them.

2.You have the most perfect ass any human can have.

3.You are an expert in cock sucking.

4.Your tits are a wonder to behold.

5.Those perfectly shaped lips of yours should be sucking on something very intimate to me.

6.Your hips, your ass, your slow walk, all beckon me.

7.My mind keeps playing back the way your perfect hips sway.

8.Your hot, sexy body is a naked weapon.

9.I thought you looked beautiful when you smile until I saw how you orgasm. Gosh! You look like a goddess in ecstasy.

10.Those lips of yours are calling out to me.

Dirty Talk in Public

These dirty phrases can turn your partner on in public and make them want to have sex with you.

1. Do you know what I would have been doing to you right now if we weren't in public?

2.I wish you can fuck me right in front of all these people.

3.Imagine us fucking in front of a hundred naked people.

4.Hey, I'm not wearing panties. Do you want us to go to the bathroom... together?

5.If you keep stealing glances at me like that, I'll drag you into that private room and fuck you against the wall.

6.If my colleagues weren't here, I'll lay you on top of this desk and fill you up till you cum.

7.Please walk ahead of me. I want to see that rounded ass of yours in those jeans.

8.Just so you know, I fucking wet right now.

9.I couldn't help but think of you holding my cock when you were on stage holding the microphone.

10.I know people are watching, but can I suck you for just a minute?

11. Slip your hands into my panties. Quick, no one is watching.

12.I know this may be a little bit inappropriate, but I just can't stop thinking about your cock inside me, right now.

13.Standing next to you in this crowd makes me want to touch your cock. May I?

14.I'm glad none of these people here know how great you are in bed.

15. Can I let you into a secret? I feel like fondling you right now.

16.Stand close to me, honey. I want to feel that cock throbbing against my ass.

17. Are there any cameras in this elevator? Because I feel like tearing off your clothes right now.

18.Can we just leave this boring event for five minutes? I'll rather be alone with you.

19.I like this bumpy bus ride; your cock keeps bumping into my ass and that's making me super wet.

20.Thank goodness these people can't see what your hands are about to do under my skirt.

21.I need to use the bathroom. I expect you will check on me in five minutes?

22.Can we just ignore all these people and bang like no one is here?

23.If you keep doing that thing you do with your eyes, I'm going to cum in my pants in front of all these people.

24.What if I go down on you right here and now?

25.This movie is boring. Can we do something fun in the back of my car?

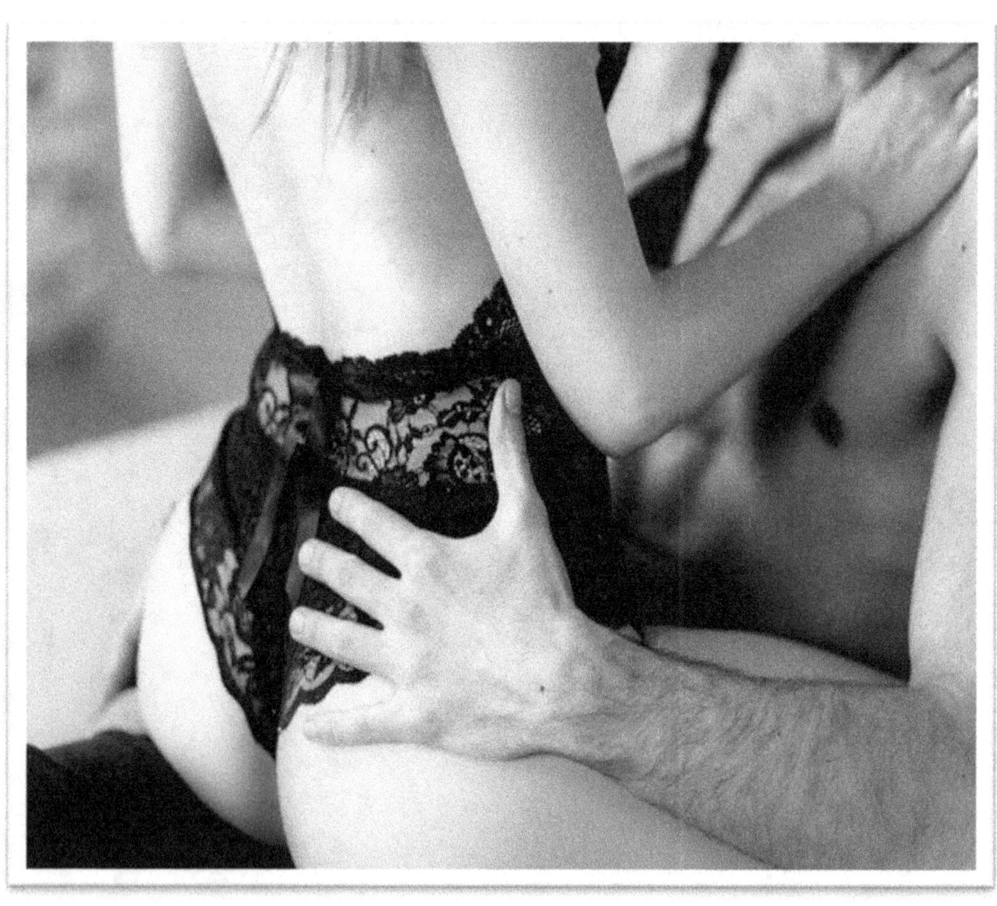

Chapter 6 Sensuous Seduction

The blinds are shut, the candlelight is gleaming, the beverages are cooling. All you need presently are some smooth moves to lure your darling endlessly from the rigors of the day and into your softening grasp. Continuously remember that no temptation is finished without some genuine kissing, Kama Sutra-style. In any case, the old writings demand that, when you've stimulated your darling with a kiss, you should be set up to catch up with other enchanting aptitudes.

The accompanying pages tell you the best way to entice in style. Pick your system and apply it with all the alluring authority you can gather. On the off chance that you decide to strip your sweetheart, strip off the layers such that fringes on respectful. If you decide on an exotic grasp, make it time-halting serious. If you treat your accomplice to some oral cherishing, give them that there's no spot on the planet you'd preferably be. Whatever you do, commit yourself, brain and body, to the occasion.

Enchantment

Enchantment can occur in the wink of an eye or the sending of an underhandedly express instant message. It can likewise be a lengthier, waiting issue, in which you can utilize the procedures appeared here. In any case, take your lead from the Kama Sutra and make temptation your top need.

The must-have-it state of mind

It's anything but difficult to jump on your sweetheart when you're in the temperament. The test comes when they're NOT in the mind-set. Perhaps they've quite recently gotten back home from work; possibly they have stuff at the forefront of their thoughts. Your responsibility is to transform them around and get them into an absolute necessity have-it disposition.

What's more, to do this, you need some hot enticement methods added to your repertoire. Attempt any of the accompanying to drive your darling wild with want: Call your sweetheart when you're only minutes from meeting them. Stimulate their feeling of expectation by disclosing to them that you're horny to the point that you need to engage in sexual relations straight away. Instruct them to get ready in like manner. Or then again, on the off chance that you need to speak to your darling's feeling of fun, have a go at luring them with sheer fun-loving nature. Challenge them to a pad battle or spruce up in their clothing and request that they strip you.

Reverse the situation

In case you're generally the one to tempt and start in your sexual coexistence, take a stab at shaking things up with some invert brain research. Tell your accomplice that you're going on a sex "detox" for a couple of days, the clue that you could be convinced to break your quick if the correct sort of allurement tagged along. You'll see a different side of them as they battle to get you into bed.

The intensity of the psyche

On the off chance that you can fill your darling's head with desire and lustfulness, you may find that their body is chomping at the bit to go before you even touch them. Take a stab at requesting that your darling depicts in detail a provocative demonstration they'd prefer to perform on you.

Sensual proposal

Pursue Vatsyayana's recommendation and enjoy some hot visit to get things moving: "... talk intriguingly of things that would be viewed as coarse, or not to be referenced in the public eye."

Playing with artfulness

Show your provocative aims by improving the bed with blossom petals. At that point, drag your accomplice into the room for some classic being a tease and caressing, so they know precisely what you have as a top priority.

Setting the mind-set

You can likewise set the disposition dial to tempting by accomplishing something exciting together, for example, slow and attractive moving. Start dressed and help each other gradually strip as the move warms up.

Grasps

A sensual grasp can take the sexual state of mind from lukewarm to torrid in the flutter of an eyelash. Little contrasts to the experience of standing and your body in a tight secure against your lover's. It enables you to put every one of the burdens and strains of the world behind you and to enter the domain of your faculties.

Outside satisfactions

The antiquated sensual writings are joined regarding the matter of grasps: they are fundamental primers to the demonstration of adoration. The AnangaRanga alludes to them as "outside delights" that "ought to consistently go before interior satisfactions." Their main responsibility is to "build up the craving... These influences and redirect the psyche from bashfulness and frigidity." Embraces are imperative to the point that they are recorded for each event, a portion of the grasps that the Kama Sutra suggests, for example, The Twining of a Creeper, ought to be "performed at the hour of welcome a sweetheart," and are expected as sexy articulations of friendship. Others, for example, The Embrace of Milk and Water, are proposed to get you boiling with anger.

Receiving the benefits

The message is truly basic: invest bunches of energy grasping in the development of sex. Embraces, strokes, snog, and nestles increase the sexual pressure, so sex turns out to be progressively dangerous when you get down to it. What's more, don't spare grasps only for sex; make them part of regular daily existence with the goal that any minute can be erotic. Embrace hi, lie weaved while you're viewing a film, and bid farewell with a hot full-body grasp.

The puncturing grasps

She squeezes her bosoms against his body in an energetic I-need you right-now signal he won't have the option to stand up to. He cups her bosoms in his grasp and strokes them delicately.

The twining of the creeper

She sticks to his body with every one of her appendages "as a creeper twines cycle a tree." She twists his head towards her face so she can look at him affectionately before kissing him delicately and exotically.

The grasp of milk and water

She sits on his lap and wraps herself firmly around him. He holds her nearby in his arms. The way that your privates are in such closeness is a genuine turn-on. Envision that is no joke "go into one another's bodies."

The squeezing grasps

Defeat by desire, he squeezes her against a divider and moves in to cover her body with his. Take a stab at pounding your hips together to get the sexual strain moving; you presumably won't have the option to control yourselves.

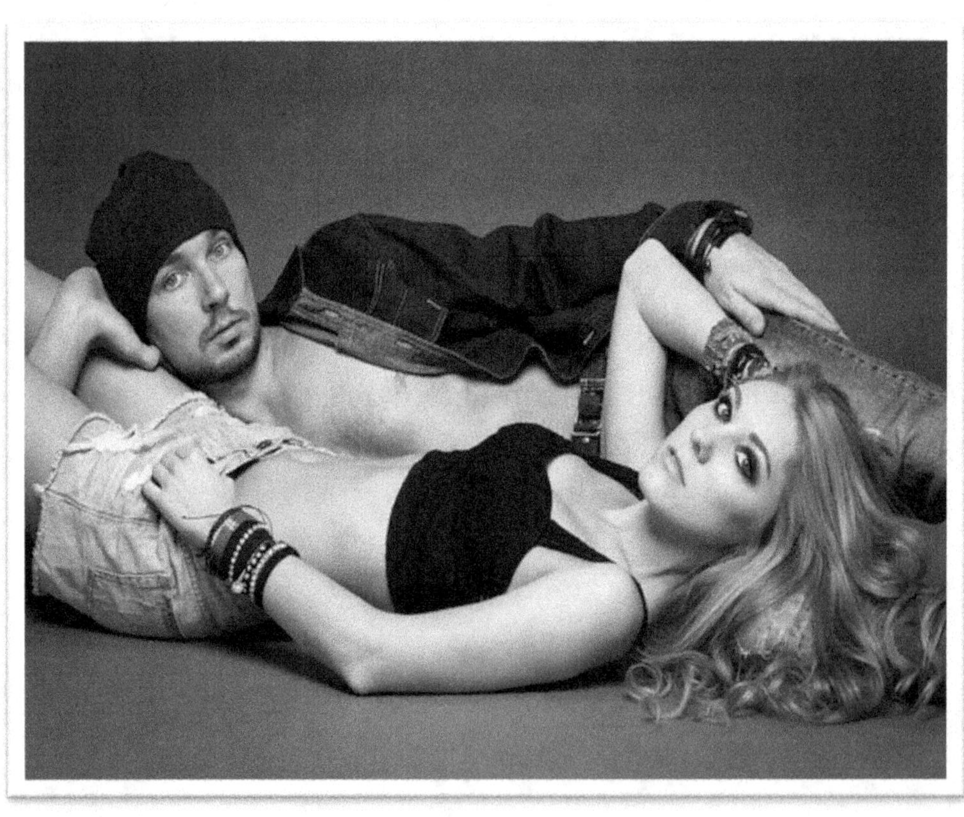

Chapter 7 Dirty Talk: Important Dos and Don'ts

Women's magazines and blogs provide us with some very important information we can't find elsewhere. We show ideas and perspectives that help people understand and cope with or satisfy them. Many women still face the shame they try to speak dirty the first couple of times.

It is possible that your man wants to speak as dirty as you do, but someone should still make the first move. It's not so hard to live it up in the bedroom, you just need some tips. Here's a few dos and you won't find the dirty talk helpful.

The Do's:-Tell him how large it is. Men are complementary suckers. Make his results, skills and body feel great. This ought to go together with what he ought to do. You should tell him what to do, how to satisfy you and how to make you feel more dirty talk.

Like anything else, you have to establish sexual confidence-before you hop into bed. It can include sex, pre-play flirting and wordplay. The good thing is that it sets the tempo and tone for the future.

The best way to dirty talk and naturally let it flow is to tell your guy how you feel. Telling him how awesome you feel inside–that's a good way to begin.

This kind of dirty talk can be a straightforward one-" Yes! "or it may be" I feel so good "or" yes, I like it, I really love it! But foolishness depends on how open and free you and your husband are. Although building trust takes time, you can eventually.

Don't try too hard or overdo it. Don't overdo it. What you saw porn stars may seem plausible, but if you yell all of the dirty phrases of which you can imagine it spoils the mood. It's better to keep it easy, but truthful than to ruin the mood.

Don't keep it up if it isn't your friend. Here sexing and word playing are critical before pre-playing. You can say if your man is playing along or resisting.

Understand what dirty speech really is, perhaps you need a guide like an eBook with everything you need to know about dirty talk. Do a little research and find the best instruction manual to guide you from the first steps to dirty speech.

Dirty talk during sex is something everybody hasn't done before. Although a majority of us want to try it - even to fantasize, very few really do.

We all know sex is an adventure, but it can also be a monotonous and dull adventure if partners do not explore new frontiers. Dirty talk will change your sexual life for the better, but there are some crucial things you can and don't have to do to keep your experience meaningful.

Your friend may want to speak as dirty as you do, but you can't rekindle things unless you try. You must start slowly; not only yell all kinds of naughty things that first come to mind.

It is best to start by quietly whispering in the ears of your partner, let him know what you want them to do or say and observe their answer. You will take it as an indication to say or do something. The first time is always a little tough, but one of you will take the initiative in order to roll the ball.

Take into account the idea of dirty talking for a few months and get to know your partner first and what kind of stuff they want.

I proposed that I spoke to my boyfriend dirty for the third month of our marriage and to my surprise it was just the sort of thing in which he was. Do not start dirty talking on your first night because it could be a turn off for some people and could be clearly disrespectful.

Practice is required to perfect dirty talk. Only through experience do you know what your partner wants to hear, what words or phrases repel him or her and what physical acts should be followed by what you say to each other.

It is also important to remember that dirty talk during sex may not be for everyone. My friend Lisa, who was a Christian reserved man, once told me that she tried to dirty talk at bed with her husband in order to spice up things but unfortunately, that had the contrary effect and caused him to immediately lose his erection.

Not only did it lead to an unpleasant circumstance, but it also led to it being called an unnecessary derogatory term. The argument here is that you must know the person with whom you are and be confident enough if you are dirty talking or not.

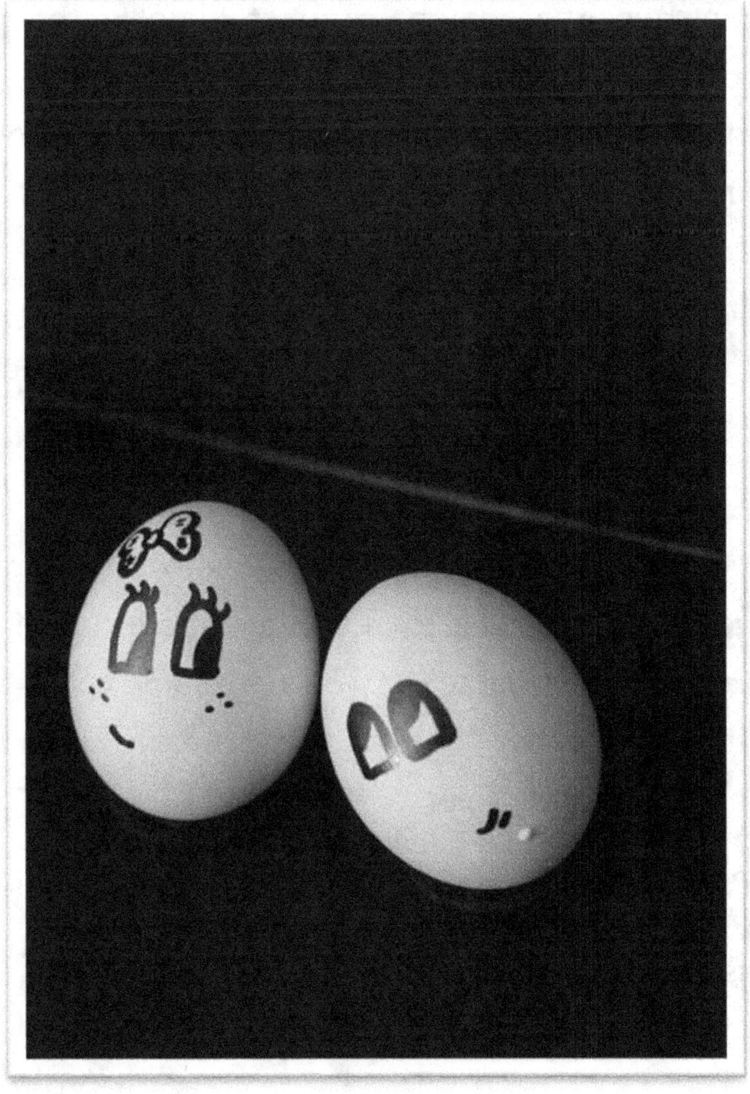

Chapter 8 Role-Playing

One of the easiest and fun ways to overcome sexual inhibitions is role-playing. Sexual role play is a game that involves acting out sexual fantasies using different roles that may be completely unlike the individuals in real life. The intensity of the play depends on the participants. You can choose to role-play using makeshift props or go into elaborate preparations complete with scripts and matching costumes for each character in the play. However, you don't need to be an award-winning actor/actress or even have any prior experience in acting to enjoy sexual role play.

This chapter focuses on the basics of sexual role play and how you can use it to improve on your use of dirty talk. The idea is to get you to assume a character that is not yours and talk like the sexy, dirty version of that character.

The Process Bring up your mutual sexual fantasies

Unless you want to take your partner by surprise and hope that they play along, it is usually better to brainstorm different ideas and scenarios with your partner. Come up with what you both think is agreeable. We all have sexual fantasies even if we don't actually want them to happen in reality. But these fantasies could be your guide to enjoying role-play with your partner. Perhaps you wish your masseur or masseuse would be a bit more daring and take things just a bit farther during your massage sessions, or you have always had an eye for one of your teachers back in college. Share those fantasies with your partner and see which ones both of you can act out.

It is crucial to do this because one partner's idea of role-playing may be too strong or kinky for the other. But when you talk things out together, you will figure out what works for both of you. In any case, it is advisable to keep an open mind and think of it all as mere fantasy and nothing more.

You can start with simple settings at first. Getting into too many details and imagination may be too daunting for you or your partner and defeat the goal of sexual role play. Start with something that can be done in a familiar setting such as your home or a nearby restaurant or bar. Select simple roles/characters and scenarios such as:

- A lonely businessman and the comforting sexy woman at a bar or restaurant.
- A pervert teacher and the naughty student in a class or the teacher's office.
- A nurse and her sick patient in a hospital bed.
- A house owner and his sexy maid in the living room or kitchen.

Dress the part if you wish

Go ahead and dress the part if it will help you to play the part more realistically. You can buy hats, wigs, and other costumes from costume shops, online, or adult shops. While costumes can add more excitement and fun to the whole idea of role-playing, they are not a requirement. Only get them if you think you really need them. Moreover, you may not have extra money to spend on costumes and props or you just want to keep things simple. Several roles require little to no costumes (a stranger at the bar, being on a blind date, and so on).

Make It kinky if you wish

Some sexual role-plays (such as officer and criminal, teacher and student, boss and secretary) are more about power and dominance. One partner (the dominant) gets to have their way with the other (the submissive). If you want to explore sexual dominance or kinkiness in a more relaxed and playful atmosphere assume the dominant/submissive roles using any character of your choice.

However, role-play is not all about power exchange. You can choose to skip any role that tends to portray the dominant/submissive attributes.

Start slow

As always, it is best to start anything new with baby steps. It may feel too unreal, ridiculous, or just plain silly to get all dressed up and act like someone else. But you don't have to dress up to start with. Playing pretend may seem like a childish thing to do, but if you let go and play along for just a little while, you may discover that you are actually turned on by the idea of picking up a stranger at a bar, for example (even if you've known this "stranger" all your life).

Even if you totally buy the idea of sexual role play, it is wise to start slowly. You can begin by sending a raunchy text or sext detailing your sexual fantasy to your partner. This can be another form of foreplay. If you are a shy person, you can use this medium to open up communication on potentially awkward or embarrassing sexual subjects.

Let your character use dirty words

There is no movie director here; it's just you and your partner. So, you don't have to feel embarrassed if you get your first few lines completely wrong. Feel free to laugh about it if you fumble or make mistakes. No one is taking a score. Just let yourself ease into character and the words will flow naturally. You may or may not know how the fantasy will end. In any case, simply let your imagination guide you into what your character will say and say them without reservation. Even if you don't like profanity or filthy words, your character may like them. Permit your character to say what they need to say to make the game fun and exciting.

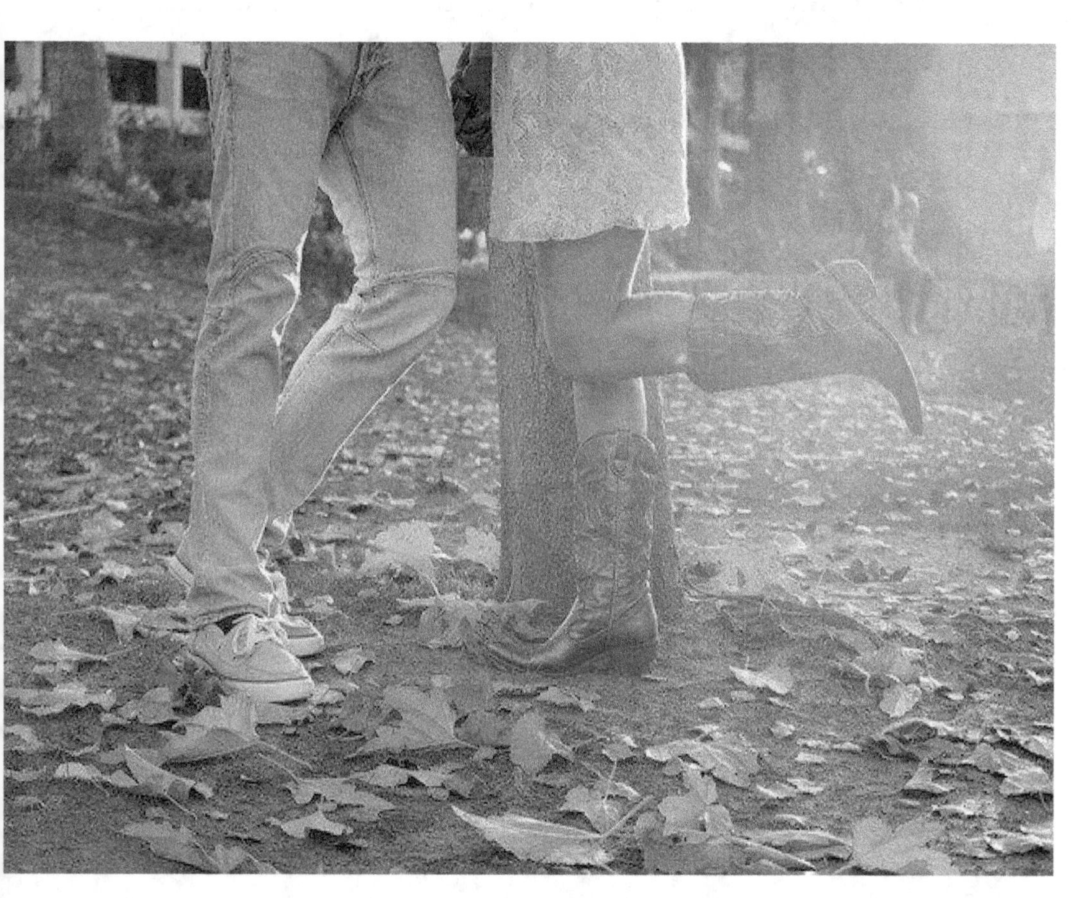

Chapter 9 Dirty Talk During The Deed

Desiring dirty talk during sex is very common for both men and women, but how do you do it? Maybe you've gotten really good at sexting and building anticipation, but the thought of translating that into actual spoken words is intimidating. You have to think about your tone of voice, what nicknames and phrases to use, and more. This chapter explores the different types of during-sex dirty talk, ideas for what to say, and how to continue dirty talk all the way through the post-coital glow.

The three most arousing dirty-talk techniques

As we've said before, any talk about the sex as you're having it is dirty talk, but there are three specific techniques you can use to really fan the flames: describing what you're feeling, taking charge, and redirecting to sexy stuff you really like:

Describing what you feel

One of the easiest ways to dirty talk is to just narrate what you're feeling in the moment. Feeling a cool tingle or throb? Tell your partner. It heightens the experience for both you and your partner when you share what's going on, and it lets them know things are going well. When you start getting close to orgasm, keep the talk going all the way through, if you can. It really turns up the heat and gets your partner excited. Depending on where you are in your dirty talk journey, you can be as general or specific as you want:

"I don't want to stop kissing you."

"My legs feel like jelly right now."

"I can't get enough of you."

"I feel so close to you."

"That thing you're doing with your tongue is driving me crazy."

"You're so good with your hands."

"You feel so big inside me."

"I love being so deep inside you."

"I'm so close, I can't stand it."

"I'm about to cum."

Taking charge

Being bossy is both sexy and gets you what you want. Both men and women often like to be dominated and told what to do, so this is the perfect style of dirty talk. Be direct with your words. If your partner wants you to be more aggressive physically, as well, go for it, but unless that's an explicit desire that you're sure about, just be bossy with your voice. Here are some ideas:

"I want you right now."

"Kiss me like you mean it."

"I want your mouth on me."

"I want your tongue in me."

"Pull my hair."

"Flip me over and do me from behind."

"Pin my arms over my head."

"I want to get on top."

"Spank me."

"Ride me fast and hard/slow and easy."

"Look at me/don't look at me."

"Say my name."

"Cum for me."

Redirecting

Using dirty talk to redirect your partner is similar to taking charge, but it's specifically for when they're doing something you aren't really feeling or they're not quite nailing a certain technique. This is common during oral sex, which can be tricky for many people, especially if they're new to giving it. Instead of just saying, "Don't do that," which isn't very encouraging, you're giving them something else to do that you do like, using your sexy voice. When they're doing something oh-so right, don't forget to affirm that, too.

"Slower."

"Harder."

"Faster."

"Gently."

"Deeper."

"Hold me tighter."

"Can you use your tongue?"

"Higher."

"Lower."

"I'm ready for you."

"Just like that."

"More."

"Don't stop."

What if the dirty talk isn't going well?

Dirty talk can be awkward, especially when you're just starting out. What if you're having sex and trying out some new words and phrases, and they just aren't landing? Maybe your partner isn't responding or you just feel really uncomfortable. Don't worry! You can make things much easier by remembering you don't need a huge dictionary of dirty things to say, and you don't have to be constantly talking. This is an example of quality over quantity. Only saying a few dirty phrases per sexy time isn't a failure, if that's where your comfort level is. Forcing more will definitely be awkward and not fun.

Are you worried that you always say the same things? Your partner isn't going to care if you fall back on classics like, "This is amazing," "I love feeling you inside me/being inside you," or "I can't get enough of you right now." If those are the genuine things you feel most comfortable saying, your partner will hear the passion and earnestness in your voice.

Also, as a note, if your partner isn't responding the way you expected, it doesn't mean they aren't enjoying the dirty talk. Maybe they are feeling self-conscious and don't know what to say back to you. After sex, ask them what they were feeling and if having them respond verbally is important, let them know. If you are the partner who isn't talking much, but wanting to let your partner know how much you're enjoying the moment, focus on sounds instead. Moaning is always welcome, though if you know your partner really wants dirty talk, consider dropping in a few swear words. These are powerful, short, and simple declarations, like "Oh, fuck," "Fuck, yeah," and so on. Phrases like, "Oh, God" will also most likely be met with enthusiasm.

Dirty talk over Skype

Thanks to the power of technology, you can enjoy romantic encounters over video chat services like Skype! This type of sex is especially valuable for long-distance couples or for couples where one partner travels frequently. It keeps them on the same page sexually and emotionally. Working through the initial awkwardness and vulnerability also strengthens a couple's trust in one another. Here's how to employ dirty talk over Skype:

Prep

It's safe to say that most Skype sex isn't spontaneous. That gives you some time to prepare what the session will look like and get ready. Maybe that means picking out your favorite sexy clothing, selecting a toy and/or lube (if you're planning on pleasuring yourself), choosing a playlist, or lighting a candle. It's also the time to think about what you're going to say. Are you going to focus on describing what you're doing to yourself or narrate what you would do to your partner if you were together? Is there a particular pet name your partner really likes?

A phrase? Putting in the effort will make the Skype sex way hotter and more fun.

Treat it like a real date

Making sure you won't be interrupted is especially crucial if you have kids or roommates. Can you even imagine how awkward it would be for everyone? Ideally, you are alone in the house with a few hours to spare. The door and windows are closed, and you're feeling comfortable. Now, treat the Skype date like a real date. Wear what you would wear when you're ready for a sexy evening in person. Focus all your attention on your partner, so put away the phone, turn off the TV, and close any other browser tabs. Imagine your partner is the only other person in the world right now.

Describe what you're doing (and what you wish you were doing)

Your voice is very important. Since your partner can't touch you, it's the most intimate connection. They can also see you, which helps, but there's something about a sensual tone that really gets the blood pumping. What are some specific things you could say?

"You look so hot right now, there are so many things I want to do to you."

"Are you ready for me to take off my clothes?"

"I'm so wet right now."

"I'm so hard right now."

"I'm kissing your neck, behind your ear, and gripping your hair hard."

"I can feel you stroking me up and down."

"I'm imagining that you're licking me right now."

"I wish I could feel you inside me/I wish I was inside you."

"I'm thinking about you plowing/doing/fucking me so hard right now."

Lots of sounds like moans and heavy breathing are great accompaniments to dirty talk over Skype. They will instantly snap you into a sexy mindset. If you aren't sure what to say, you can always read some erotica out loud. If you like to write, you can even write your dirty talk beforehand and read it, so it's totally original and your partner knows it came from your mind.

Dirty talk after sex

Dirty talk doesn't have to stop once the sex is over. It's a great way to keep the intimacy and communication going, and provide feedback on what you really liked. It's also a good time to bring up things you would like to try the next time things get hot and heavy. Here are some examples:

"I'm still weak in the knees."

"My head is still spinning."

"I'm not sure I can stand for a while."

"I loved those sounds you were making."

"It was so sexy when you...(said/did this particular thing.)"

"Mmm, I love that I can still taste you."

"We have to do that (thing you really liked) next time."

"I'm going to be thinking about that all day tomorrow."

"I wish we could just stay here like this forever."

What not to do

We've talked about dirty talk techniques and given you some examples, but is there anything you should not do when trying it out with your partner? There are three main rules to follow:

Don't laugh at your partner

Dirty talk can be awkward, especially when it's brand-new. You may feel relatively comfortable with your tone and words, but your partner may still be getting used to it. They may come up with something that's cheesy or funny, and you're tempted to chuckle. Resist. Laughing will make your partner feel really dumb and they'll clam up. They might not want to try dirty talk ever again. Instead of laughing, suggest other things they could say or a name you like, so they can try something else.

Don't say things you're not comfortable with

As you read about dirty talk and start experimenting, you might bump up against words or phrases you really don't like. However, your partner might respond to them in a really positive way. Maybe you hate calling your partner a "bitch," but they really like it, and they want you to get even more aggressive. It can be tempting to not talk about how uncomfortable you are because your partner is happy. This can be very harmful to your relationship. You'll feel false or worse. Because you're so uncomfortable, you won't be able to fully enjoy the sex and your partner, and that's bad for both of you. Talk to them. You can find a compromise.

Don't rush in

Dirty talk has many layers and tones. Most people like to ease into it, even if they have an idea of how extreme they would like to go. This is a good idea because it lets both you and your partner discover your limits and what you really like. Rushing in can be overwhelming and create some uncomfortable or even disturbing situations that paint dirty talk in a bad light. Being a bit cautious and careful is especially important if you and your partner have not been together very long. You're still establishing trust. Just take things slow. It's about the fun and excitement of going on the journey, and not reaching a set destination.

What about dirty talk and role-playing?

As you were reading this chapter, you might have wondered why we weren't bringing up role-playing. Don't worry, that is actually getting its own chapter. Dirty talk is an essential part of fantasy and role-play, though it can take a while to get comfortable if it's unfamiliar to you.

Main takeaways

There are three very arousing types of dirty talk during sex: describing what you're feeling, telling your partner exactly what you want, and redirecting your partner to try something else.

If you feel awkward trying dirty talk and it doesn't seem to be going well, you can fall back on words or phrases you are really comfortable with, or focus on making sounds instead. You don't need to break out something fresh every time.

To have good Skype sex, have an idea about what you're going to say and do, and treat the event like a real date. If you're pleasuring yourself, be sure to describe what you're doing for your partner and detail what you wish you could do to them.

Dirty talk can also be a part of your after-sex experience. Talk about what you really liked, what you want to try next time, and just enjoy each other.

The only things you should not do when dirty talking is laugh at what your partner says, say things you aren't comfortable with, and rush the process. These three no-no's paints dirty talk in a negative light.

Sexual Roleplay Ideas

Here are a few sexual roleplay ideas to help stimulate your imagination and get the ball rolling. You are welcome to tweak them to suit you and create your own dirty dialogues along with it. You can use the dirty phrases in parenthesis as part of your sex dialogue.

1. Play the role of a firefighter who just rescued your partner and is rewarded with sex. (Dirty phrase: "You

saved my life. The least I can do is to offer you my dick/pussy.")

2.Play the role of a cop. Your partner is trying to get wriggle their way out of a speeding ticket. (Dirty phrase: "The only to get out of this is to please me.")

3.Play the role of a prostitute who's just having sex for the cash. (Dirty phrase: "Show me the cash and I'll give you good pussy/cock.")

4.Pretend you came for a sleepover at your friend's and snuck out to have sex with your friend's sibling. (Dirty phrase: "Shhh... come have a taste of this cock/pussy before someone sees us.")

5.Pretend that you are a client getting a massage from your partner who is a masseur or masseuse and is willing to give you a happy ending. (Dirty phrase: "Could you go a bit lower... lower still, yeah... that's the spot.")

6.Pretend to knock on the wrong hotel room door but the stranger who opened up (your partner) invited you in any way. (Dirty phrase: "Never mind, I could use the company of someone as gorgeous as you right now.")

7.Play the role of a landlord who's come to collect their rent, but your partner can't pay, so they end up paying in kind. (Dirty phrase: "I'm gonna fuck my money's worth out of you tonight.")

8.Play the role of a yoga instructor teaching your partner how to stretch and bend over. (Dirty phrase: "Nice and slow... that's it. Now bring that sexy ass of yours over here.")

9.Play the role of a boss who is about to have sex with his or her employee on the desk. (Dirty phrase: "I see you've been striping me naked with your eyes all day. It's time to turn this office into our sex haven!")

10.Both of you should assume the role of angry partners in a rough sex session.

11. Play the role of a tour guide with a strong accent. Let your partner listen to your dirty talk with a different accent.

12.Recreate the roles of your favorite porn stars from a porn scene or novel.

13.Play the role of a naughty maid trying to have quick sex with the house owner before the wife shows up. (Dirty phrase: "I'll be in the kitchen... I've got no pants on. Hurry!")

14.Pretend to be a dance teacher and seduce your student (partner) through your movements. (Dirty phrase: "Place one foot ahead of the other and move your hips this way. Gosh! You look so sexy in that pose!")

15. Play the role of a hooker trying to get a one-night stand. (Dirty phrase: "I'm free for the whole night. Would you like to do something fun and sexy?")

16.Play the role of a pizza guy who gets a blow job in place of cash. (Dirty phrase: "I'm sorry I don't have any cash at home. But I'm sure we can figure out some other more interesting way to pay?")

17. Pretend is your first sex as husband and wife on your wedding night. (Dirty phrase: "I've been waiting for this moment all my life. I can't wait to finally be inside you / have you inside me!")

18.Play the role of an artist and paint your nude partner on a canvas. (Dirty phrase: "You have the curves of a god/goddess.")

19. Play the role of a shy virgin having sex for the very first time. (Dirty phrase: "Promise to be gentle with me tonight, would you?")

20. Play the role of an innocent person who is completely naïve about sex. Let your partner teach show you how to have sex. (Dirty phrase: "Is that what an erectpenis/aroused vagina looks like? Oh... I see.")

21. Pretend you are a student who's trying to seduce their teacher for better grades. (Dirty phrase: "I might not be good at algebra, but I can tell from the way you look at me that you want to have a taste of me, don't you?")

22. Pretend that you are a hypnotist who has hypnotized your partner. Command them to do whatever you wish. (Dirty phrase: "You will suck my cock / eat my pussy when I instruct you. Nod if you understand me.")

23. Play the role of a nurse and bathe your "sick" patient (your partner). (Dirty phrase: "If you would step out of your robe. Good boy/girl. Now relax let me take good care of you.")

24.Pretend that you are a striptease and give your partner a lap dance. (Dirty phrase: "Do you like it when I bend over and shake my ass like this?")

25.Play the role of a cab driver and have sex with your client in the back of your car. (Dirty phrase: "Your destination is still a bit far. I suggest we stop here for a while, grab a quick bite and have a quickie.")

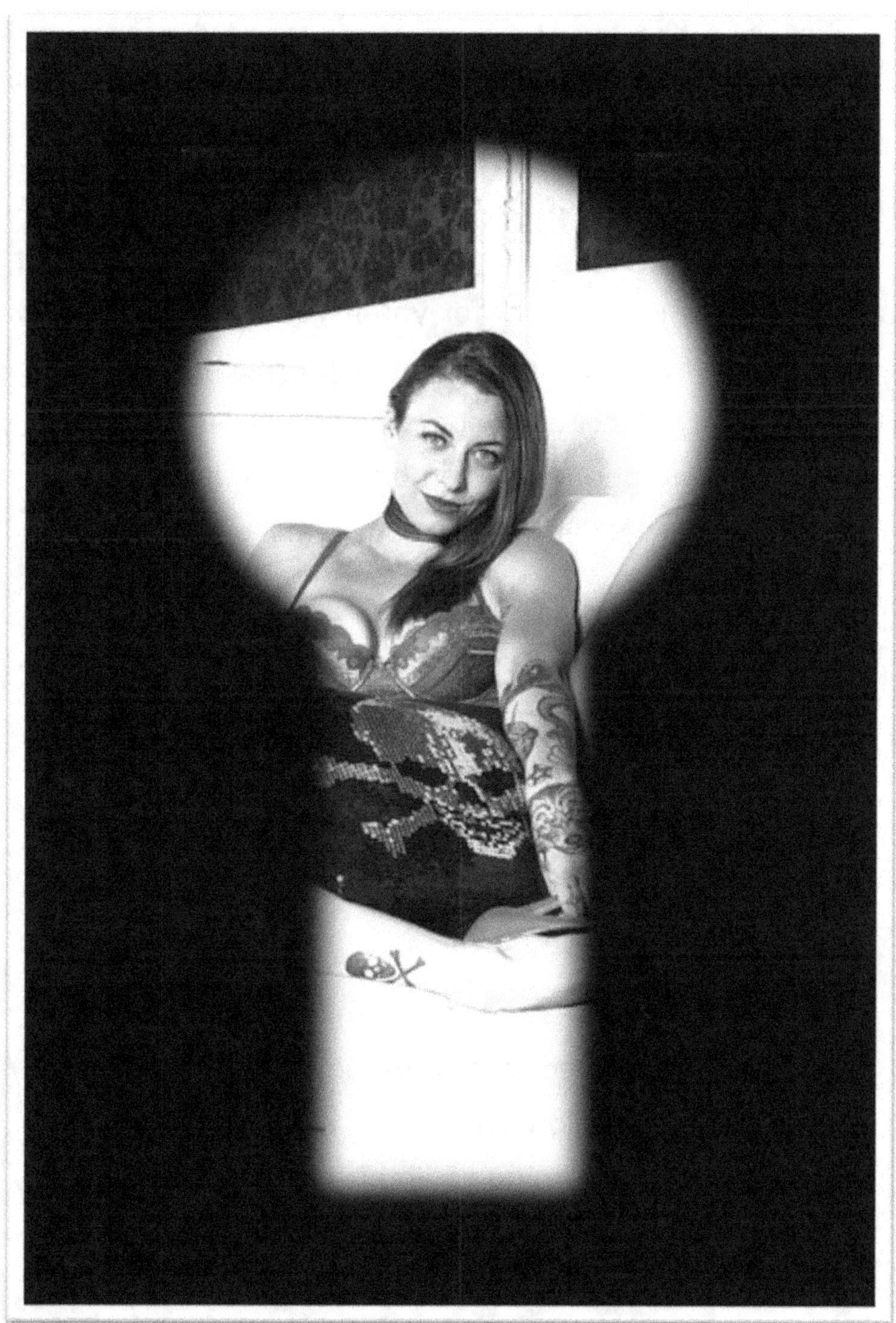

Chapter 10 Phone Sex

Whether your partner lives with you or you are in a long-distance relationship, you can take advantage of technology to spice up your sex life with phone sex. Phone sex can also work for you if you don't want to have other forms of sex with your partner just yet or if you simply want to try something new. Although the idea of having phone sex can be exciting, it may be really awkward when you actually want to try it out for the first time.

Having physical sex or even masturbating alone is a lot easier because then no one else is aware of what you are doing. But having to possibly masturbate (it's not compulsory to do so) with another person hearing and maybe even seeing you through video requires a different level of boldness.

To make phone sex a great and sexually exciting experience, you need to give up being self-conscious and intentionally allow yourself to respond to the sounds and sight coming to you from the other end. Also, remember to have a conversation instead of a monologue. Phone sex is not a hypnotic session. Both partners should share what they are doing, imagining, and feeling.

Sex on Call

The process

Plan ahead: Spontaneity is great when it comes to sex, but sometimes you may call your partner at the wrong time. To avoid this, set a date and time that is most convenient for both of you. If you are in the mood for sex while your partner is having a bad day, calling them at that time may ruin your mood. Also, if your partner is the shy type, it may be a good idea to get their minds prepared on time before you pounce on them with your sexy talk on the phone.

Put yourself in the mood: Feeling awkward or tensed before your call will likely ruin the mood. Do what you need to do to get in the mood before the call. You can have a glass of wine, watch short porn, read a romance or porn novel, or even dancing. Dressing sexily and lying down for a while can also put you in a sexy mood. You can also dim the lights, play your favorite soft music, bring out some sex toys (if you use them), and gently caressing yourself before making the call.

Make the call: There is no one correct format for phone sex. However, once your partner is on the phone with you, it is better to start slowly. Talk about other things for a few minutes before gradually broaching the subject of sex. Make your voice soft, low, and don't be afraid to moan. You can use heavy breathing too as long as it comes naturally. Don't force yourself to sound sexy.

Talk about easy things: You don't have to directly bring up sex even if both of you know the call is about sex. Ease into phone sex with simple topics that can easily spiral into hot sex. The following lines will give you an idea of how to do this.

1. What are you wearing?

2.It's cold here. I wish you were here.

3.This bed is just too wide for me alone.

4.I'm lying on your side of the bed and playing with my hair.

5.I wish you were right here beside me.

6.Tell me what you are doing with your hands?

7.Tell me what you would have done to me if I were there with you now.

Talk dirty: Once the mood is right, escalate into dirty talk. Since they are not physically with you, your dirty talk will have to be descriptive. Both of you can describe:

·What you are doing: give your partner a vivid description of how and where you are touching yourself, how you look, what you are playing with, and so on. You can say things such as:

1. I'm playing with that whip you bought from an adult store for our first role play.

2.My fingers are teasing my cock as we speak.

3.I'm touching my tits and my nipples are so hard.

4.I'm playing with my undies… they are coming off soon.

5.I'm getting really wet and horny.

6.I enjoy listening to your sexy voice. It's making me hard/wet.

7.I'm running my fingers through my hair.

8.I'm jerking off to the sound of your sexy moan.

·What you are imagining: Tell your partner something you remember from one of your great sex you had, what you would have loved to be doing with them, or what you would want them to do to you. For example:

1. I'd like to hug you real close and feel the warmth of your soft skin.

2.I'd like to kiss your neck, lips, and tits ever so softly.

3.Remember how you took me from behind the last night we had together? Now, take me again!

4.I'm touching myself and thinking how great your hands feel all over me.

5.Touch your clit and feel my warm breath on your pussy.

6.I can imagine how rock solid your cock will be now. I want to stroke it and suck on it with my wet lips.

7.I can tell you are soaking wet. Imagine me eating out that wet pussy.

8.Put one finger in your mouth and imagine it's my cock in there.

·How you feel: It is important to let your partner know the effect of the conversation on you. Describe how you are feeling physically and emotionally. You can moan loudly, scream (if you have to), or breathe deeply. Let go of all inhibitions and allow yourself to be fully expressed. You can say something such as:

1. The sound of your voice is making my heart beat faster.

2.I feel like exploding when you sound like that.

3.Say that again... please. If feels so good to hear you say that.

4.You are making me quake with that moaning sound.

5.I feel like appearing right there with you.

6.I feel sexy when you call me your little girl.

7.I feel like kissing your lips now!

8.Oh my God! I'm coming!

Masturbate if you feel like it: If you choose, you can masturbate while talking with your partner and let them listen to all your moans, or you can engage in mutual masturbation. But this is completely optional. It is okay to skip it if it doesn't feel right or appropriate. It is also important to keep in mind that phone sex may not always end in orgasm. Only one of you may climax or both of you may fail to climax and that is okay. Orgasm is not the main attraction of phone sex. However, if you have climaxed and your partner has not yet reached orgasm, don't end the call or keep mute. Continue to describe how you feel, what you want them to do, and so on.

Finish the call: You can end the call at any time both of you choose. You must not reach orgasm before ending the call. Also, you shouldn't end the call just because you've both climaxed. You can stay on the line for as long as you both choose and talk chit chat a bit.

Talk about it afterward: Don't be shy to talk about the phone sex afterwards. You can even text them how great it felt. Compliment them either on call on through text and make them know that you are looking forward to another great phone sex. Keeping shut about it afterward may suggest that you are uncomfortable, or you feel guilty.

Sex on video call

You can take advantage of different technologies (FaceTime, Skype, Zoom, and so on) to have sex "face-to-face" over your devices. Seeing what your partner is doing, their reaction to what you are saying, and the expressions on their faces, can add to the arousal, especially for men.

To avoid frustration and disruptions that can kill the mood, make sure that your internet signal is strong enough for video calls or else simply stick to phone sex.

Sexting

Sexting is using digital messages to convey erotic intents. Thanks to technology, people can now send naughty messages back and forth without having to deal with the uneasiness that comes with saying these words face-to-face.

You can use sexting to gauge a potential partner's openness even before dating them or having sex with them. However, sexting techniques range from subtle to direct methods. It is always a good idea to begin sexting with subtle messages that can pass as flirting. If the other person responds positively, you can then up your game to messages that puts them in a sexy mood. Finally, you can sext messages that make them want to have sex with you so badly.

Sexting can be done using text only or inserting photos, memes, emojis, and emoticons. Get creative with your messages and make them unique. The following examples are just to give you an idea of what sexts look like. It will make more impact if you adapt your sext to something you and your partner share or experience. For example, instead of just sending, "I can't stop thinking of your sexy ass," you can personalize it to read, "I can't stop thinking of your sexy ass in those red yoga pants." Or "Those pants hug your ass so tightly I feel like touching myself."

A good sext is usually short and stimulates sexual imagination. Even when you use sexual innuendos, keep it brief. If you can make room for humor, that will be great too.

Go through the examples below and let your creative juices guide you into creating customize sext messages for your long-term partner or someone new you are trying to have sex with.

Beginner sexting examples

1. Guess what? I'm at work thinking of you and touching myself right now.

2. Your hot ass/legs dominate my thoughts all day.

3. What part of my body is your favorite?

4. I can still feel your warm lips on my cheeks.

5. I really need you right now.

6.Can we do it in the shower tonight?

7.I'm soaking wet right now. Can you come over for a quickie?

8.Next time, I'll lick more places on your hot body.

9.Your cock/pussy makes me go insane.

10.You went down on me and I lost all my senses.

11. You. Me. Under the sheets... pure heaven!

12.I love how hard you gave it to me last night. Let's make it even rougher next time.

13.I love how you take charge of my body.

14.I want you to dominate me tonight.

15. This early morning's quickie was delicious. Can we continue tonight?

16.I get goosebumps when I think of your hands in my pants / up my skirt.

17. You look so sexy and innocent when you giggle.

18.I don't feel like having my bath just yet. I love the smell of you on me.

19.Whenever you pass by, I get a boner. Can you help me fix that?

20.Let's do something freaky tonight. Got any sexy ideas?

21.I want to have dinner off of your body tonight.

22.I need your naked body on mine right now.

23.Picture this in your mind: you and me, naked under my sheets.

24.Let's have a mixed wrestling match tonight. No count-out or disqualifications. Don't worry; I'll be gentle when I slam you on the bed.

25.URGENT! Can you please help me with five synonyms for FUCK?

Advance sexting examples

1. What crazy place should we fuck next time?

2.You have no idea how hard you make me want to fuck you.

3.Your ass is so sexy it deserves an Instagram page.

4.My dick/pussy still feels lusciously sore from yesterday's pounding. You sure know how to handle me.

5.I can still taste your sweet cum on my lips.

6.I'll like you to cum all over my tits tonight.

7.Come straight to bed after work. There's a wet pussy waiting to be fucked!

8.Three things occupied my mind all day: your sumptuous boobs, succulent lips, and wet pussy!

9.Thinking of the sound you make when you cum makes me want to cum in my pants!

10.I'll let you cum in my mouth if you let me sit on your face tonight.

Creative sexting examples

1. A sexy surprise awaits you tonight… *insert wink emoji*

2.I've been thinking of your *insert peach emoji* all day.

3.I'll love to do this tonight… *insert sex position GIF*

4.Your ass is so *insert hot/fire emoji* it makes my dick *insert raindrops/sweat droplets emoji*

5.*Insert bondage GIF* Tonight will be fun!

6.I want to *insert tongue emoji* your *insert peach emoji* right this minute.

7.Me when I saw your naked boobs last night *insert head exploding GIF*

8.*Insert eggplant emoji* Free services tonight. *insert wink emoji*

9.*Insert image of a man proposing* with a meme caption: When she says, "Cum in my mouth."

10.*Insert an image of a breathless woman or woman fanning herself* with a meme caption: When he asks, "How would you like to be fucked tonight?"

11. Tonight was exceptional. Thank you! *insert heart and worship hands emoji*

12.Meme caption: You: smooching my cock/tits. Me: *insert fainting image*

The Use of Photos

Although photos and images can increase sexual arousal, men are generally more visual than women. If your sexual partner is a man, they will find some of the ideas here very stimulating. That doesn't mean women can't be turned on by raunchy photos. However, a man needs to first set the mood right through flirting, sexting, or sexual innuendos before jumping to sharing explicit photos.

Sext with photo examples

1. Thinking of you while I do this... *insert a photo of you masturbating or one you downloaded.* (If you use a downloaded photo, crop off the face. You want your partner to imagine you and not someone else.)

2.Stepping out of the bathtub... *insert a sexy photo of you all wet!*

3.Going shopping with absolutely nothing underneath... care to join me? *insert photo of a see-through dress*

4.I'm in bed, wearing only this... *insert photo of sexy lingerie*

5.I'm bending over the sofa where we fucked last night. Wanna see? *insert sexy photo*

6.These will greet you when you come home tonight... *insert photo of boobs*

7.*Insert photo of hot legs* Come spread them!

8.I accidentally fell into the pool just now. Please call 911. *insert photo of you or someone clothed in a wet sexy dress*

9.I keep fantasizing about this... *insert photo of erect cock*

10.Would you be so kind as to teach me how to do this... tonight? *insert porn photo of sex position*

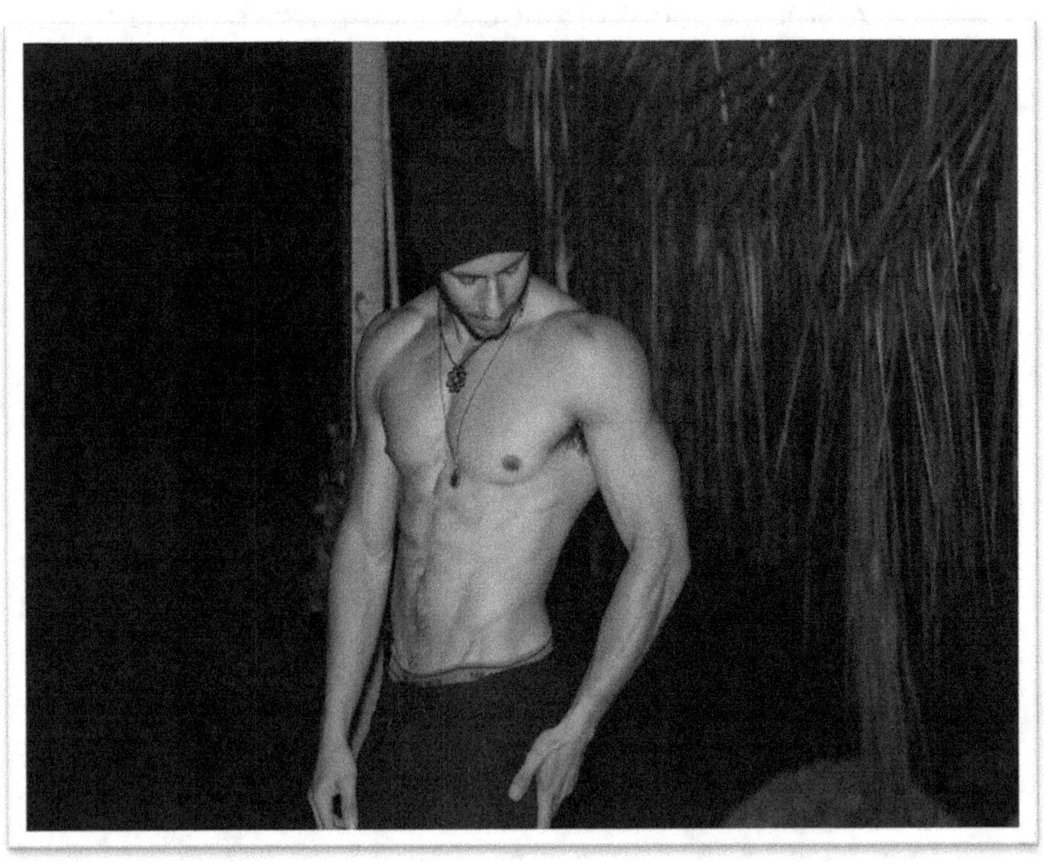

Chapter 11 Overcoming Shyness to Keep the Dirty Talk Going

Talking is easy enough most of the time. We've been talking ever since we could form the words and understood what they meant as a kid. Talking is easy, but dirty talking? Well, that's something else altogether. Even the most talkative, chatty, outgoing, friendly personalities hit a speed bump when it comes to playful pillow talk. There's bound to be a naughty word or two that can make even the most sexually confident person turn bright red with embarrassment. Why do we react this way? Other times we have no problem voicing our opinions, even when nobody else wants to hear them. Yet dirty talk can reduce you to a flustered, tongue-tied ball of nerves. That's because sex has always been more about "doing" and less about "talking".

Talking dirty is like stripping off your clothes in front of a new partner. You're nervous and wondering what they think or how they feel. Every word or phrase that you utter is like another piece of clothing being taken off, and all the while you're wondering if they like it.

Are they turned on by it? Or worse, is it putting them off? Do they find it sexy when you do this? Do they want you to stop? With so much to think about it's no wonder building our carnal confidence verbally is not the easiest task. If you've never done something like this before in front of your partner, the sudden use of vulgar words might catch both of you off guard or even shock you.

Overcoming Shyness Step 1 - Practicing on Yourself

Overcoming shyness is going to be tricky for a lot of people, so before you start trying out some of your newfound dirty vocabularies out on your partner, a better idea would be to practice on yourself first so you can get the feel of it and get comfortable with the idea of saying this out loud. Pick a couple of words or sentences to start with, and then practice talking dirty to yourself as you masturbate. Don't worry about feeling silly, no one can hear you anyway. As you masturbate, talk dirty to yourself to heighten your arousal. Focus on the pleasure that you feel and blurt out how you honestly feel. Simple phrases like "Oh yes, that feels so damn good" is already off to a good start. It's better than staying silent anyway and the more you practice repeatedly talking to yourself, the less awkward it becomes with each practice session.

Overcoming Shyness Step 2 - Imagination

Once you've become comfortable with Step 1, it's time to take it to the next level. The second step to getting over your shyness is to imagine you're now having sex with your partner while you masturbate. Do everything that you were doing in Step 1, except this time you're going to add an element of visualization into the mix. If you're the man, visualize that you are now sliding your hard penis into your partner's vagina as you slip it between your fist (don't forget to use lubrication). As you visualize and slide fist up and down your penis, imagine it's your partner on top of you and you're telling her "Baby, your pussy feels so good and tight". If you're the woman, visualize that your man is sliding his penis in and out of you as you use your fingers (or a vibrator) to do it. While you do this, imagine your man is on top of you right now and tell him "Your cock feels so hard inside me. That feels so good".

Overcoming Shyness Step 3- Honesty

Now, words like "good" are considered basic level dirty talk, but it is a good place to start practicing with as you work your way up to the more explicit stuff. Dirty talk talks confidence, and if you don't have it, you need to work on it first or it's going to sound uncomfortable and forced when you try to do it with your partner. With dirty talk, the one rule you need to remember is this: The greater your description, the better the impact. Be as descriptive as possible to make it good for both of you. The easiest way to do this is to vocalize all the sensations that you feel. If her pussy feels tight, tell her how tight it is and how good that feels. If your man feels nice, hard, and thick inside you, let him know how good that feels. Describing the sensations you feel in an honest, raw way so that it hits home and doesn't feel like you're faking it. For example, don't describe your partner's penis as "thick" if it doesn't feel that way and you both know it. Honesty is going to be the best approach in this instance.

Think of the best way to describe each sensation that you feel with honesty. Think about your partner and what they like. What do they want to hear that is going to stroke their ego and boost their confidence. If your partner is worried about his size but you love the way he feels, then tell him you love how he fits you perfectly. Is your partner self-conscious about her body but you find it incredibly sexy? Tell her how just looking at her is enough to bring out the animal within you.

Overcoming Shyness Step 4- Think Positive

Most people are too hung-up over the notion that dirty talk is cheap. That it's not something "good girls" or "good boys" would do. You might expect that from low-grade porn movies but that's about it. If you're hoping to become a lot more erotically eloquent, then you need to get over this idea that sex is dirty or unclean and so is talking that way. Sex is part of what it means to be human, and trying to deny that fact is like denying a part of yourself. Your sexual persona is only one part of who you are. It doesn't define you. Just because you like it dirty in the bedroom, it doesn't mean that's who you are in real life.

Our bodies and our genitals are not dirty. Words like penis, breasts, balls, vagina, boobs, cock, and pussy, those are not words to be ashamed of. They are nothing more than terms used to describe the various parts of our bodies and treating them like a shameful thing is only feeding into the stigma around dirty talk. Take off your clothes, stand in front of the mirror and look at your body. Look at your genitals, touch them and say the words out loud. Describe what you like most about what you see. If you think your breasts are your best feature, then say that out loud in front of the mirror. Tell yourself "My breasts are incredible", or "My nipples are perfect, small, perky, and just the right size. My breasts are a nice, big, generous handful and they drive my man wild.". Focus on only positive body image talk when you're doing this exercise. Learn to love your body for what it is. There's no need to compare them to anyone else.

Overcoming Shyness Step 5- No Judgment Zone

The bedroom is the one place that should be free of all judgment. Couples should treat this as a safe space they can be open and honest with each other about their innermost kinky thoughts without fear of being shunned or judged by their lover. Remember, healthy sexual communication is good for your relationship and keeps you both on the same page. Refrain from criticizing your partner when they bare their thoughts, even if what they say happens to take you by surprise and absolutely refrain from rebuking your lover when they're trying to tell you how they feel. Honesty is a key theme in this chapter, and it is what you should keep coming back to. Be honest and respectful. If what your partner said maybe felt a little too dirty for you, let them know and work out a compromise you can both agree with.

Great sex involves giving and taking. Both partners need to be actively involved. Dirty talk needs to be reciprocal, not just one partner doing all the work and dominating the conversation. It's important to take turns vocalizing how you feel so there's an opportunity for both partners to get to know each other in a deeper sense.

Overcoming Shyness Step 6- Build Your Vocabulary

As children, we were taught to read a lot to develop our vocabulary and this same principle can be applied once again to what goes on behind closed doors. There are more than enough words that exist today describing sexual experiences and genitals. Erotica novels, porn movies or video clips, slangs and sensual films should be treated as a source of information and give you an idea of the kind of words you would like to use yourself. If you want to describe intercourse with words other than f***ing, alternative words include boning, shagging, screwing, bumping, grinding, and more.

Using the word vagina not your cup of tea in the dirty talk department Try alternative words like pussy, or cheery pop. As for adjectives, there's juicy, mouthwatering, succulent, moist, yummy, or luscious. As for the penis, words like cock, dick, jackhammer, love muscle, joystick and more that could be used as descriptors.

Overcoming Shyness Step 7- Laying Down the Ground Rules

It's easier to come out of your shell when you feel secure enough to do it and that's what ground rules are for. If this is something, you're both new at and trying for the first time, setting some rules and boundaries helps to maintain a level of respect. Your partner may be open to the idea of being called a "naughty little slut" but you may not be open to being called a "cockwash" just yet. For couples who are worried about dirty talk sounding cheap, ground rules are going to help them get over those obstacles.

Be mindful of each other's boundaries as you acclimatize to this entire experience. Carrying out your sexual fantasies can be incredibly hot in bed, but only if you're both on the same page about it. Boundaries are not meant to serve as restrictions, but rather to give you a sense of security so you both know when not to go too far. It helps you keep the entire experience as enjoyable as possible. Boundaries are there for your benefit in the beginning. If you want to test them or push past them later once you've gained more experience, you can, but only if both of you are comfortable with the idea. Like sex, this is a two-way street and both parties must give equal consent or it's not going to be as enjoyable as it should be.

Overcoming Shyness Step 8- Experiment with Voices

Play around with the different voices you might want to use. Does telling your partner what an animal they are in bed sound sexier in breathy whispers? Or when you're moaning or screaming their name out loud?

Experiment with both options to get a feel of which one sounds better to both of you. Perhaps you weren't a screamer before and this is unveiling a different, sexier side of you that turns your partner on. Be unpredictable and challenge yourself to try something new. Surprise your partner so they can never predict what's going to come out of you next. Are you going to moan his name in a sultry voice while he's pounding into you hard? Scream how good it feels when his tongue is tantalizing your clit? Growl in her ear her how incredibly good and feels as you vigorously thrust in and out? One of the most exciting aspects of dirty talk can be catching your partner off guard to keep the anticipation alive.

 Once both partners are comfortable with the dirty talk being a regular feature in the bedroom, try coming up with your own secret love language as you get creative with the words you use. This kind of talk is meant to excite you and titillate you, and if the current coital vocabulary is not doing your desires justice, feel free to invent your own. There's something intimate about sharing a language no one else but the two of you know, and it can bring you closer together as a couple.

The Cycle to Overcome Shyness

Dirty Talk for Shy People - The Best Time to Do It

As if we didn't already have enough to be anxious about, now we need to add anxiety over dirty talk into the mix. The common themes that pop up among couples who have never attempted this before and are too afraid to try are:

- They worry that they are going to freak out their partner.

- They worry that their partner is going to see them in a different light if they start introducing this in the bedroom. What if they think you're too promiscuous? Or sex-crazed? What if they don't respect you anymore if you talk like this? What if they think you're a pervert?

They worry they might get carried away and say something that crosses the line. There's an episode of Sex and the City that's a good reference point for such a scenario. When Miranda was dating a man who liked to talk dirty, she was shy and nervous at first about trying it out. Once she got over her initial hesitation though, she opened Pandora's box and never saw the man again.

You're not alone in the fears and concerns you have. Men and women have concerns about dipping their toes into this territory. It's like dipping your toe into the pool to test the waters. Only once you dive in, you realize it wasn't so bad after all. Dirty talk is the same thing. It is exciting and seductive and lauded as an easy way to give sexual consent or tell your partner you're ready without disrupting the flow. Grabbing your partner as you place one hand behind their head, gaze hard into their eyes and say f**k me is an incredible turn on for some couples. It is an intimate and private language that bonds two people together.

Even the most verbose individuals can find dirty talk a challenge. It's easier to see words on paper than you imagine yourself saying them out loud. Trying to make yourself sound sexy when you don't feel sexy can make you feel foolish. When is the right time for dirty talk? When the moment feels right to you. There is no good and bad timing, it depends entirely on the context of the situation. You never know when you might suddenly be in the mood for sex, and trying to fix a specific time to talk dirty is only going to make it feel forced, monotonous, and routine. Surrender yourself to the moment and go with the flow, sometimes the most exciting sexual encounters are the ones that you least expect.

Other Tactics to Help You Shed Your Fears

Still feeling shy despite going through the steps above? That's okay, you're nervous and that's understandable. You're not sure how you feel about all of this yet, and you're worried your partner is not going to respond the way that you hoped. What might help you ease into the process as you gauge their reaction would be to describe what you want to do to them or what you're doing. If you're too nervous to do it in person, there's always phone sex or texting to get the ball rolling.

Tactic 1 - Naughty Text Messages

Surprise your partner by sending them a naughty text message in the middle of the day. There they are, going through a normal work routine when suddenly their phone lights up with a text from you and they see I can't want to put your breasts in my mouth and suck on those sweet nipples hard. It catches them off-guard and puts a smile on their face because they immediately start to visualize what that would feel like. They'll respond with something equally naughty in return and before you know it, you can't wait to rush home and start having your way with each other.

Doing it over text takes some of the anxiety away that comes with doing it in person. You feel "safer" somehow behind the confines of your screen and the idea of an on-screen rejection feels better than a face-to-face one. Plus, when your partner responds well to your attempts over text, that gives your mind the proof that it needs. It tells you your partner is enjoying this as much as you are. Once you know they like it, your confidence starts to grow from there as the fear of rejection dissipates. Knowing that they find this just as much of a turn on as you do makes it easier to transfer all this naughty talk from text to in-person when you see each other later after all the teasing that has been going on all day.

Naughty texts build the tension before the sexual encounter so that by the time you're ready, you're so wild with desire for each other the sex is amazing right from the start. Here are some examples of easy text conversation starters you could use to start teasing your partner with:

•	I can't wait to see you tonight. I know exactly what I would like to do to you ;)

•	I had a naughty dream about you last night. How about we make that a reality tonight?

•	Take off your underwear by the time you get home or I'm going to rip it off.

•	I'm in the mood to make you scream tonight. You should be prepared ;)

•	I've got a sexy little surprise for you tonight honey ;)

•	I'm having a hard time concentrating at work today. I can't stop thinking about all the dirty things I want to do to you tonight.

•	I just got out of the shower, you should be here (have a sexy photo ready to send with this one if you're comfortable with it).

•	What should we have for dinner tonight? Besides your pussy/cock in my mouth.

- My body still feels deliciously sore from what we did last night. You are an animal.

When coming up with naughty little snippets to send to your partner, a good rule of thumb would be to think about something specific from the last time you had sex and then describe that and tell them what is on your mind. "I can't stop thinking about yesterday when you grabbed me and lifted me up onto the kitchen counter. I didn't know sex in the kitchen could feel that good. You should be here right now so we can do it again", is one example of a text you could send to stir your partner's sex drive again. Should you want to drive then even wilder, think about sending them sex-laced text messages before or after you masturbate. This is a more advanced move for couples who are already comfortable with some dirty talk going on every now and then, but it is certainly effective at building your confidence and sexual openness.

Tactic 2 - Reading Erotica Together

Have you ever thought about reading erotic novels together as a couple? These books can be surprisingly helpful since they are packed with vocabulary that is meant to stimulate your imagination, given that no pictures are available. Notice the words and language that is being used in these novels and the way the author has described the scenes that are taking place so there is no mistaking that the couple in the novel is definitely about to have sex. Talk to your partner throughout the process, see what they think about it. Which sentences or passages did they find most arousing? Which words sparked something in their genitals and wake it up as they were reading it? Tell them about which ones stirred something within you and made you feel a spark of desire as you were reading it. Ask them if you should try taking it to the bedroom and role-play what it would feel like to say these words out loud.them about which ones stirred something within you and made you feel a spark of desire as you were reading it. Ask them if you should try taking it to the bedroom and role-play what it would feel like to say these words out loud.

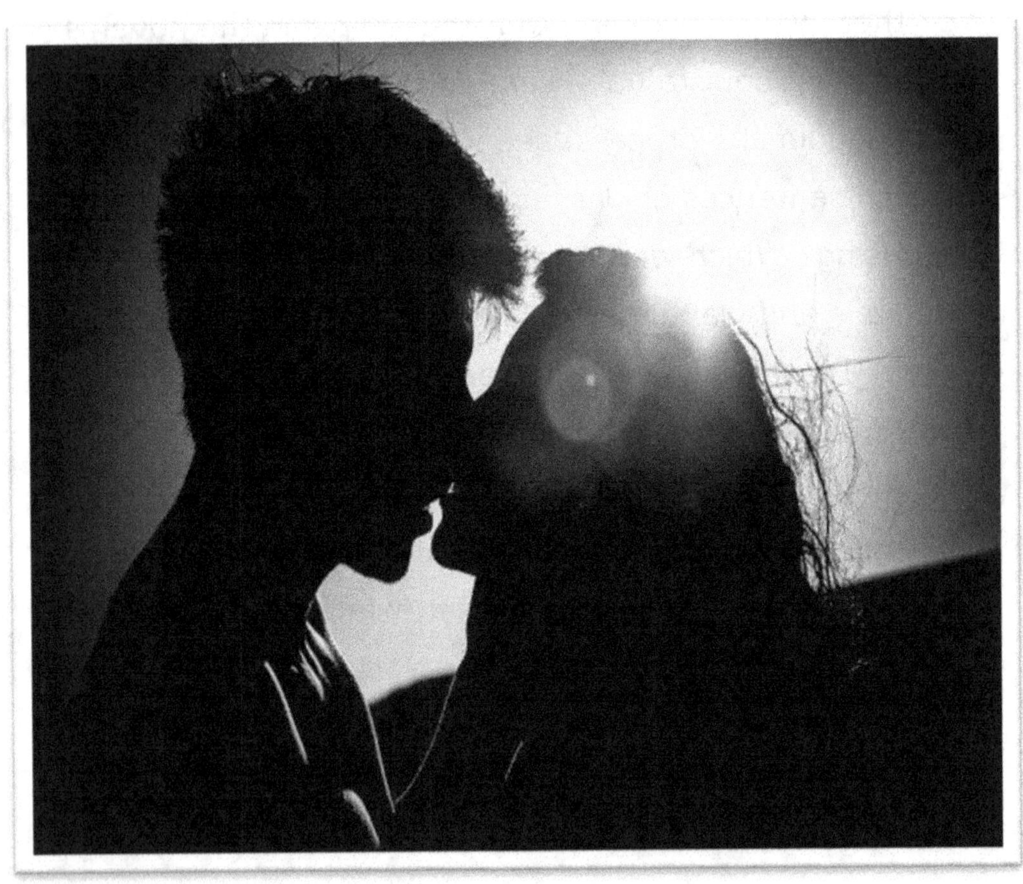

Conclusion

Sex is a beautiful thing! It can be more exciting if the people involved let loose and express what they want and like. It can be more attractive if the people involved are not ashamed to openly lust and feel lusted after. And it can be more beautiful if the people involved want to devour each other (not literality, of course) and are not afraid to say so!

One of the greatest and most priceless gifts you can give to yourself and your partner is your unabridged, uncensored, authentic, and fearless self. When you permit yourself to be you, you will be pleasantly surprised at the level of pleasure you can give and receive. But beyond that, you increase the chances of improving your overall relationship with your partner. Great sex can, indeed, improve the quality of your relationship, health, and even boost your self-esteem.

Remember that you don't have to go from being extremely shy to pro overnight. Forcing yourself to talk dirty will only make you sound awkward to yourself and your partner. Take baby steps. Start with the most comfortable and easy words. Rehearse your lines as if you are going to act in a movie. Allow yourself to say those words that resound in your head. You can practice in front of a mirror if you like. Become comfortable with hearing yourself say the words before telling them to your partner.

Remember though that dirty talk is not something you should just jump into without letting your partner know. Of what use is an attempt to spice up a relationship if it only makes things awkward? You wouldn't want to say things that will embarrass you or your partner so it is best that you talk it over with them.

Using dirty sentences does not also mean that you should end up giving weird names to your sexual organs or your partner's. Some people abhor some words and you try to find out what counts as a taboo for your partner. The secret to sex is not all in the position you use or the words you speak to one another. It is in relationship. This is true whether you are in a friendship that is sexually laced or you are in a relationship that is committed or just dating and experimenting. The secret to a great sex life is the knowledge of who you are and what you are shooting for together. Sex is but a mere fraction of a relationship. It is but an expression.

You can unleash this kind of dirty talk in person or via text, but it's clearly easier by text as you have time to think. Smoothly stringing together dirty talk in person takes a little practice, but the benefits it offers make it more than worth the effort. More importantly, you're only going to get better with practice. Who cares if it doesn't come out as flawlessly as you'd like? Chance are good that your partner will still be turned on, which is all that matters.